"In a self-effacing, 'Dr. Heal Thyself' style, Bi[...]
the journey from victim to victor. I will recon[...]

> *Dr. Ken Pepperdine, Chiropractor, Nanaimo, British Columbia*

"This book is an inspiration for all, and especially for those with health challenges. Bill and Denise are exceptional people. Their friendliness, warmth and positive attitude are appreciated by the many people who are fortunate enough to meet them."

> *Patricia Kongshavn, PhD, Immunology,*
> *former Professor, McGill University, Montreal, Quebec*

"An exceptional book to read and keep as a personal guide and reference. Bill and Denise willingly share some of their personal life experiences and well researched knowledge to help us all gain our own path to optimal health. An opportunity of a lifetime!!!"

> *M. Tobler, RN (retired), Cobble Hill, British Columbia*

"I understand Dr. Bill's health challenge because of some of my own. In 1943, age 6, I was hospitalized with TB of my right hip. They kept me in a whole body cast for the next six years in the TB solarium (hospital). Then in 1948, they fused my hips with a bone graft from my left shin. The body cast worsened the inverted breast bone I was born with, so I had major chest surgery, age twenty. My surgeon told me that without the surgery, I'd be dead within three years as I had chest asthma as well. He and I were both happy I made it through the surgery. His first such surgery had died on the operating room table. I was his second such procedure. Pain from movement and weight gain from inactivity have been my constant battle. In the last four years, I have read all three of Dr. Code's books. They have helped me reshape my life and health immensely. His last book, *Winning the Pain Game,* is the easiest to read and understand, even with my grade 8 education. I regularly use all of his '10 Choices for Chronic Illness.'"

> *Frank O'Neill, Nanaimo, British Columbia*

"I consider Dr. Bill Code my wellness coach. Together with his wife, Denise, Dr. Code has made a significant impact on my overall health and wellness through his book *Who's in Control of Your MS* and his personal recommendations. As a person living with MS for 37 years, the importance of managing a chronic illness effectively cannot be overemphasized. Dr. Code's writings and lectures have provided me with valuable information on how to maximize my wellness through proper diet and informed supplementation. I attribute my good health, including weight control, pain relief and sleep management to Dr. Code's straightforward and well-researched recommendations."

Christopher R. Fortune, M.A. Graduate Certified Executive Coach,
Victoria, British Columbia

"Your book served as a reminder that there is always more we can do for ourselves to improve our health. My hope is that people not just read your book, but that they put into action the things you suggest."

Wendy Bowen, Physiotherapist, Duncan, British Columbia

"I'm feeling great. My neurologist actually said I've improved from last year. Thanks for your support, Bill."

Jock MacDougall, Vancouver, British Columbia

"Bill and Denise are both very committed to easing the pain in people's lives. They have worked very hard to create *Winning the Pain Game* and have produced an informative, easy-to-understand, useful book for anyone who suffers from chronic pain."

Mary Cook, Duncan, British Columbia

"Have read your book – it is excellent....Thank you for publishing a book that covers alternative ways to deal with this chronic disease – it is not fun to have."

Carol Foster, Administrative Government Assistant,
Victoria, British Columbia

"I want to congratulate you for daring to pursue a healing path even though that meant straying far from what you learned in medical school. I find that a great many people come to Integrative Medicine because they first realized its potential in their own life. I trust many are finding benefit in applying what you have learned. Certainly your vitamin D chapter makes perfect sense, and I think conventional medicine will rapidly catch up to what you are saying in the coming years."

Larry Willms, MD, Sioux Lookout, Ontario

"Words cannot express our gratitude to you for writing such an excellent book. It has been really helpful."

Cathy Preyra, Ottawa, Ontario

"I loved the book. It gave me confidence and it reinforced that I was doing things right for my health."

Suzi Ness, Alaska

"I just finished reading your book *Who's in Control of Your MS*. I found the book very helpful in providing alternative therapies for MS."

Kelsey Hoffo

"How many books have been written on alternative healing! Now and then one appears which actually offers something new and helpful. *Who's in Control of Your Multiple Sclerosis* is one of those rare, easy-to-read exceptions.

But there is more here than empathy and an encouragement to 'take charge' of one's life. Dr. Code carefully outlines a comprehensive set of tools by which chronic sufferers can help minimize their afflictions and, hopefully, reverse their conditions. *Who's in Control* is packed with coping and healing strategies, such as the chapter on dietary supplements that could serve by itself as a stand-alone primer. This chapter is something even healthy individuals would find helpful, along with the closing section on Dr. Code's 10 Choices for Chronic Illness."

Paul Rothe, Victoria, British Columbia

"I have read your books but when I finished the last book you gave me, when we were at Edgar and Ruby's, I was so overwhelmed by your story I cannot help but write to you. Your thoughts, your pain, the frustration, and how you have worked your way to what you are today is truly an amazing victory.

Years ago when I first heard you had MS, you were in my thoughts very often. I prayed that you might be able to help carry on and use your talents.

Thank God, that has happened with much effort on your part, you didn't give up and I marvel at how energetic you are.

I pray for your future years that you can keep on doing what you are doing now.

Bill and Denise, you will always be in my thoughts and prayers!"

Tina Harder, Saskatoon, Saskatchewan

"Dr. Code,

You have made a difference in my outlook after my diagnosis of M.S. You have answered so many questions about the condition. I now know which vitamins and minerals to take and how to live my best life.

Thank you for your book, which I have read in detail so I feel more confident about my future."

Diane Needleman, RN, Key West Florida

A New Look at Relieving Pain and Enhancing Healing & Health with Integrative Medicine

For some doctors, pain and chronic illness are their specialty. For Bill Code, after contracting MS, it was his daily reality. But being the scientist and the man he is, Bill was not going to accept the dismal medical verdict without checking all the information—even the avenues he had been trained to discount or ignore. When he did, he found life-changing answers, and he shares them in this book.

Integrative medicine has steadily reached new levels of respectability thanks to the efforts of doctors like Andrew Weil, MD, and now Bill Code, MD. Highly motivated by his own illness, Bill, and his wife, Denise, a registered dietician, threw themselves body and soul into the study of pain and brain issues from an integrative approach. They were continually surprised, even astounded, at just how many options were available that they had not previously learned about when they studied the literature of their respective fields.

Of course, they had to sort through a vast amount of information to find the material that was supported by rigorous scientific evidence. But find it they did. The result was that Bill started to experience a greatly improved quality of life, including less pain, less fatigue, less brain fog, less falling, and fewer muscle spasms. The ultimate outcome was the restoration of his health.

Integrating all they learned, Bill and Denise created *Winning the Pain Game*. It is a practical map through the complementary but still non-traditional medical part of the journey to recovery and optimal health. It presents solid and specific suggestions for enhancing the immune system and the body's natural mechanism for dealing with pain and illness. It reveals a multitude of ways you can minimize the likelihood of contracting illness or disease and maximize your body's innate ability to protect and even heal itself. And it shares the many resources Bill and Denise found to deal with pain and enhance relief.

Becoming sick is not something to wish upon anyone. However, for the Codes it was the stimulus to looking outside the box and the creation of a book destined to help many avoid pain and debilitating illness through integrative medicine.

WINNING THE PAIN GAME

July/07

To Jennifer,

To Health!

Bill Code MD

Welcome to Cowichan
Valley.

Winning the Pain Game

*The surprising discoveries
of a pain relief doctor in his search
to relieve his own chronic pain*

DR. BILL CODE, MD & DENISE CODE, RD

WORDS
·OF·
WISDOM
PRESS

Words of Wisdom Press
30765 Pacific Coast Hwy., #266
Malibu, California 90265
1-888-746-1593
www.drbillcode.com

Publisher's Cataloging-In-Publication

Code, Bill.

Winning the pain game : the surprising discoveries of a pain relief doctor in his research to relieve his chronic pain / Bill Code & Denise Code. -- Malibu, Calif. : Words of Wisdom Press, 2006.

    p. ; cm.

    ISBN-13: 978-0-9787463-0-8
    ISBN-10: 0-9787463-0-9
    Includes bibliographical references and index.

    1. Chronic pain--Treatment. 2. Pain--Alternative treatment. 3. Analgesia. 4. Patient-controlled analgesia. I. Code, Denise. II. Title.

RB127 .C63 2006
616/.0472--dc22

Cover and Book Design: Patricia Bacall
Copyeditor: Brookes Nohlgren
Book Consultant: Ellen Reid
Cover Photography: Bettina Antle

ACKNOWLEDGEMENTS

Thanks to our family: Alice Code, and of course, our three children—now all in their twenties—Laura, Brian, and Warren. We also thank our Book Shepherd, Ellen Reid, for her patience, wisdom, and guidance in bringing this book to fruition. Thank you, too, to Ellen's team: Laren Bright, Patricia Bacall, and Brookes Nohlgren—it was a superb team effort! Thank you to the Capital Region Chapter MS Society of BC and key people with the MS network: Jeanette Hughes, Christopher Fortune, Jan Yuill, Ann Muir, Bonnie Pashak, Brenda Adam-Smith, and Todd Abercrombie. Special thank you to Mary Cook for her assistance with the manuscript, Bettina Antle for her photography talents and Terri Smith for her contribution on aromatherapy in the "senses" chapter. And finally, we thank the scores of people we have met on this journey, whose questions and quest for health inspired us to write this book in order to reach out to many, many more people looking for answers.

DISCLAIMER

The authors and publisher wish to express their hope that the contents of this book will help many on the road to health, happiness, and a long, vibrant life. However, no information in this book is presented with the purpose of diagnosing or prescribing. One may use this information in cooperation with one's physician in a mutual desire to build and maintain health. In the event that one uses this information without his doctor's approval, he is prescribing for himself. This is his constitutional right; no responsibility is assumed on the part of the author, the publisher, or the distributors of this information. It is not the purpose of this book to replace the services of a physician nor is it the purpose to guarantee any medical or nutritional preparation or the effectiveness thereof.

DEDICATION TO
DR. DONALD WINSTON PATY
(1936-2004)

I first met Dr. Don Paty in July 1996 when he diagnosed me with multiple sclerosis (MS). He was just back from his own health crisis of 18 months—a bout with lymphoma cancer, treated with a bone marrow transplant. Few things can modify our outlook or "wake us up" more than a brush with our own mortality. When I found out I had MS, Don made a tremendous difference in my life. His teaching, patience, and wisdom greatly accelerated my education and deepened my understanding of the subject, and I truly appreciate his generosity while treating me as a colleague.

Paty's father was a medical missionary and Don certainly brought his parents' idealism to the single-minded goal of unraveling the puzzle of multiple sclerosis. He displayed dedication, organizational skills, and the ability to identify a problem and really deal with it. After receiving his MD from Emory University, he did his neurology training at Duke. Then, after a research fellowship in Newcastle-Upon-Tyne, England, he joined the Neuroscience Department at the University of Western Ontario, London, Canada, and worked closely with his colleagues to establish a multiple sclerosis research clinic at the London Health Sciences Centre. When I visited Dr. Ali Rajput, Neuroscience Chief at the University of Saskatchewan, I learned that Dr. Paty was considered one of the best MS neurologists on the planet—high praise from such an experienced academic neurologist.

In 1980, the University of British Columbia, Canada, recruited Don to become head of Neurology and he held that position until 1996. In June 2004, Dr. Paty was awarded the Canadian Meritorious Service Medal for his pioneering work with his colleagues in the use of MRI for the diagnosis and treatment of MS. He was also honored numerous times for his research and service by medical associations throughout Canada, the United States, and Britain.

Colleagues and patients will sorely miss Dr. Don Paty. I dedicate this book to him with great fondness and admiration.

—Dr. Bill Code, MD

"The doctor of the future will give little medicine, but will interest his patients in the care of the human frame, in diet and in the cause and prevention of disease."

—*Thomas A. Edison*

CONTENTS

PREFACE

A Few Words from Dr. Bill Code, MD

Where were you at age 42? Or, where do you see yourself at that point in your life? I was at the height of a challenging and hectic career in medicine, looking forward to continued success and satisfaction in my work. I was enjoying my family and the community in which I lived. Life was indeed good. But at 42 I was diagnosed with multiple sclerosis and could no longer work. My life turned upside down.

As a typical workaholic male, I had wrapped my self-esteem into a nonstop commitment to helping others. All of a sudden my reason for being, as my family's breadwinner, was taken away from me and I was forced to realize that I had seriously neglected the development of my own self-worth. Reeling from the huge blows to my self-image, I learned the hard way that what really matters in life is personal relationships—those with your partner, family, and close friends. I was shocked to discover that professional support is incredibly rare within medicine, and during my first year away from work only three colleagues even contacted me. This lack of connection was a great disappointment to me during this time of illness and stress. I went from being the chair of the Medical Advisory Committee in our local hospital to being described as "unsafe" to work in any part of anesthesiology!

In an effort to regain my privileges at the hospital, I was forced to get legal assistance from the Canadian Medical Protective Association. The hospital's Medical Advisory Committee was split on the issue; it seemed that the surgical specialists sided with the remaining anesthetists in wanting to prevent my return to medicine, while most family practitioners and other medical specialists could see my side of the situation.

The anger and pain over this issue between friends and colleagues became intense. Thus began my own personal, dramatic, and life-changing journey in dealing with illness and striving toward health.

Fast forward … during the latter part of 1997, I attended a conference in Vancouver about complementary and alternative methods of healthcare for MS, focusing on helping people slow down or learn how to tolerate many of the MS symptoms. This was a whole new experience for me. I was part of a large group of folks with multiple sclerosis, at all stages and all ages. Compared to many, I felt incredibly lucky because I was still able to walk, albeit with a limp. More importantly, I realized that many others were seeking new options in their own process with this chronic illness, and that opened the door for me to consider that I might be able to actually control my MS. The impact of feeling that I wasn't a total victim was deep and profound!

I finally realized that until I could let go of the anger and "poor me" complex, I could not move on. *I* was the only variable that could be changed in this scenario. It took me more than a year to appreciate that I was the only one who could have a significant impact on my multiple sclerosis. After some time, I began to benefit from empowering myself to make a difference for *me*. My wife, Denise, and I quickly mobilized to examine what we could do together (she being a dietician) to look at diet changes we could implement or particular nutritional supplements that might make a difference in my chronic illness. We spent three years searching, experimenting, discovering … and over time I realized that this body of new information could address and help more people than just those with MS. It could also help those with other chronic disease, chronic pain, and auto-immune disease.

I must confess, if someone had told me I would be concerned about nutrition or personal training skills in my late 40s and 50s, I would have said, "Not bloody likely!" But, I would have been both wrong and short-sighted. I now believe that Denise and I can help people more by sharing what we have learned together than by my practicing medicine (Anesthesiology). Thus, we happily give to you the many ideas and solutions that can have a significant impact on your road to health or on the health of a loved one.

None of these recommendations are risky or harmful, nor are they intended to replace your neurologist, internist, or family physician. Rather, these choices can and do complement traditional medical therapies; that is, these choices can be implemented along with any treatment prescribed by your doctor. My only request is that you get to know more about your illness than your family doctor does and that you keep an open mind while keeping your healthcare practitioner in the loop. You are empowering yourself as you proceed on this journey, and I wish you well.

"Let food be your medicine and your medicine be food."

—Hippocrates

A Few Words from Denise Code, MSc, RD

Life was wonderful! Bill and I had completed our educational goals, raised three healthy children, and achieved significant milestones in our careers. When we moved to the Cowichan Valley in 1992, we left the hectic pace of city life and career demands to slow down, play more, and enjoy our family on the west coast of Canada. The future stretched out before us, promising an abundance of goodness.

We decided to move to a home with acreage, which led to us collecting an assortment of farm animals including cows, pigs, sheep, and horses. Our two youngest children joined the 4-H Club and Bill became an assistant leader. Through our travels with 4-H, we also became interested in emu farming (large, flightless birds originating in Australia). As wife, mother, farmer, bookkeeper, and occasional dietician, my life was fuller than ever!

Then, something began to change. I didn't know what it was, but Bill seemed edgy and impatient and our children often found themselves at loggerheads with their dad. I was the buffer, trying to soothe hurt feelings, but it seemed that nothing the kids or I did was right. Tension mounted in our household, and anxiety increased. Besides the mood changes, Bill always seemed tired. He frequently napped, saying, "I must have the flu." I was becoming exasperated but attributed the fatigue to his busy medical schedule and being on night call. Meanwhile, there were farm chores, household duties, and childcare responsibilities to attend to.

When the neurologist told Bill that he had multiple sclerosis, I felt somewhat relieved that he did not have ALS (Amyotrophic Lateral Sclerosis, or Lou Gehrig's Disease). Finally, I could better understand what was behind all of the turmoil we had been experiencing. The relief was quickly followed by fear and overwhelm. How would I cope with my husband's major illness, as well as the needs of our children and our farm? What would the future bring? How would Bill's illness progress? How would we support our family? It was, without a doubt, the most painful and difficult time of our marriage. Many a time I secretly shed tears, driven to the breaking point. I fantasized about living on a deserted island, free of stress, free of care. But I wasn't leaving.

Much of this time is a blur, and I was definitely operating in survival mode. When Bill first became ill, I felt vulnerable because I did not have regular work. Fortunately, I was able to obtain full-time work as a clinical dietician at the hospital. Certainly the new source of income helped ease some of my angst over finances. My job also gave me an outside focus and an oasis from the turmoil in our family life. I was grateful for the opportunity to continue to grow professionally and to work with so many wonderful colleagues.

At this time, Bill began investigating other ways to improve his health and energy. He tinkered with diet choices, and initially I was a bit skeptical. Although I was trained as a dietician and was used to reading about clinical tests and applying nutritional recommendations, I was still quite traditional in my outlook. But once Bill began using emu oil and eliminating wheat from his diet, he actually made some dramatic improvements … and I got excited. He and I realigned and grew much closer as we explored new possibilities and a new philosophy for healthier living.

Prior to Bill's illness, we were both "conventional" healthcare providers, believing in the medical model of diagnosis and treatment (i.e., drugs). But during this time, our points of view changed regarding the healthcare models in which we had been trained. We realized that we no longer believed that drug therapy was the first line of defense, and we admitted that all scientific research is not necessarily as credible as we once thought. I recognized it was time to leave the hospital and its traditional practices to commit time, energy, and a growing passion to reshape our ideas and practices for a new model of recovery and wellness.

Once I left my job, Bill and I began to work even more closely together to share the wisdom and information we had gathered. We were both busy presenting health seminars. Bill focused on helping people with chronic illness and MS, as well as on educating audiences about the health benefits of glutathione enhancement. My seminars were mainly for individuals with heart disease. And though both of us were presenting valuable ideas and powerful information that were new and certainly not from mainstream medicine, we became frustrated at reaching only a limited number of people at a time. This book is the result of our commitment to helping a greater number of people take charge of their health journey and transform their lives on the road to recovery. We know that those with chronic pain, autoimmune diseases, MS, memory loss, and depressed mood will benefit from the solutions we offer. We are delighted to share our wholehearted belief in the value of seeking out alternative health practices and practitioners, in the power of food to heal and restore, and in the ability to regain hope as you embrace body/mind/spirit in a vital and wholistic approach to optimal health.

"Do no harm." —Hippocrates

Welcome to the Road to Recovery

Remember when life was slower, when families ate home-cooked meals together and outdoor play and fresh air were the norm? How times have changed! Today, we live in a fast-paced world and have stress-filled lives. We rush through each day, often with little regard to how our diet, exercise habits, work, leisure time, and environment affect our health and well-being. In fact, we take so much for granted; that is, until we get sick and suddenly realize the profound importance of feeling good.

The original focus of this book revolved around our experiences of living with and positively impacting Dr. Bill's affliction with progressive multiple sclerosis. Both of us know firsthand how ill health can bring challenges. We also know that health recovery is possible, and we are convinced that everyone needs to be proactive. If you have good health, preserve it as much as possible through healthy food and lifestyle choices as well as nutritional supplements. Do what you can to learn about the body/mind/spirit connection. If you have an illness, educate yourself as much as you can about your illness and know that you can make choices that will help you recover. This, too, we know from our own experience as well as from watching others.

Over time, we realized that the safe and alternative suggestions we've gathered and applied through research, extensive training, and clinical experience are not limited to treating MS but are also useful for all kinds of poorly resolved clinical issues such as constant fatigue, auto-immune challenges, and chronic pain. As you dive into the material, you'll also discover valuable tips to optimize your health on all fronts, including anti-aging strategies and tools to support more balance in body and mind.

Quick Overview

Winning the Pain Game covers everything you need to know to optimize your health, right now. We will help you understand how to detoxify your body as well as learn what the best nutritional choices are in foods and food supplements (including our personal favorites: brown flax, finely ground; DHA from fish oil or krill oil; and whey protein isolate), with special chapters dedicated to a wide range of subjects including vitamin D, glutathione—the master antioxidant within our body—and calcium and magnesium for those of you with reduced activity and increased risk of osteoporosis.

Why would anybody apply or swallow emu oil? The reasons for using this anti-inflammatory product will be outlined, including all the current research. A number of other natural products will be discussed including ginkgo biloba, ginseng, and other potent energy tonics. Whenever these items are used, we want everyone to consider the risk-benefit ratio. If, after this consideration, it seems a reasonable way to proceed, then go for it! We also recommend that you avoid or minimize foods to which you know you are, or may be, sensitive.

Exercise—why bother, or better yet, why work with an enlightened physical or personal trainer? We will describe how it is often possible to retrain both our balance as well as our backup motor nerve pathways. Fortunately, the Master Designer gave us five times as many motor nerve pathways as we typically use in a lifetime. Concepts of energy production and fatigue problems will be reviewed.

The final chapters discuss in depth the personal, psychological, and soulful journey we made with our experiences as "MS person" and "MS caregiver," respectively.

By the way, we have not attempted to replace our medical colleagues. Neurologists are absolutely key for diagnosis and their expertise and, in conjunction with general (family) practitioners and other specialists, use all pharmaceutical choices to the best of their abilities. Neither have we focused on particular herbal or other alternative medications, knowing fully (Bill is an experienced and formerly academic anesthesiologist) the potential negative interactions between these and drugs of today. Just be aware, consult your healthcare practitioner, and use common sense as you build your own health plan.

Dr. Bill's Journey

We suggest that you consider Dr. Bill's multiple sclerosis a prototype or example of most any other auto-immune or chronic illness. "Auto-immune" means that a segment of our white blood cell population is making an error and chewing away on a particular body tissue. Auto-immune illnesses make up by far the majority of our chronic health problems and include rheumatoid arthritis, lupus, psoriasis, Crohn's disease, ulcerative colitis, iritis, scleritis (and perhaps also glaucoma), type 1 diabetes, many skin eczema conditions, Sjogren's syndrome, ALS (Lou Gehrig's disease), fibromyalgia, thyroiditis (high and low), sarcoidosis, and quite possibly significant parts of our kidney, liver, and cardiovascular illnesses.

Healing in our bodies, whether from chronic pain or from acute injury, always follows the inflammation steps: redness, swelling, heat, and loss of function or pain. Several of *Dr. Bill's Top 10 Supplement Choices for Reversing Aging, Reducing Pain, and Improving Energy and Brain Function* (see page 107) will be helpful to modify or fine-tune the inflammatory response. As Dr. Andrew Weil describes in his anti-inflammatory discussions, these foods can also be powerful assists of our general health, well-being, and even anti-aging.

Beginning Your Journey

Many self-help books exist on nutrition and the optimal use of health-care practitioners. Why did we write this one? Our goal is to restore hope where many have lost it, by relating our personal struggle with a devastating illness first by "talking the talk" and then by "walking the walk" of health recovery. Our goal is not to diagnose, treat, or cure your illness, but instead to improve your quality of life—in other words, get your life back. Once your quality of life is recovered, many of the same solutions and practices in this book can and will enhance your quantity (length) of life too. Of course, you will continue to work with your healthcare practitioner, whose ongoing role it will be to diagnose and treat any acute exacerbation of your chronic illness or any new illness.

In summary, this book provides a two-part discussion. Part One is about reducing chronic pain and fine-tuning the body's inflammatory or healing response. Part Two is about Dr. Bill's journey with a demyelinating auto-immune illness, multiple sclerosis. In Part One, you will find pearls of wisdom to help you have less pain, less fatigue, less brain fog, less falling, and less muscle spasm. In Part Two, whether you suffer from MS, auto-immune diseases (including chronic fatigue and fibromyalgia), or chronic pain or illness, you have in your hands a viable road map through the complementary but still non-traditional medical part of your journey on the road to recovery and optimal health.

We are honored to empower you to take charge of your personal well-being while you continue to work with your healthcare practitioner. Begin your journey with an open mind and an open heart. It is only through the teamwork of mind, body, and spirit that we can minimize our suffering and optimize our well-being and health. Now, let's get started.

Guidelines for Using This Book

Winning the Pain Game is organized into two main sections:

Part One: The Road to Recovery is a general handbook of innovative and important concepts and suggestions for everyone, specifically folks interested in reducing pain, increasing energy, increasing strength, improving immune function, and enhancing brain function (e.g., problem solving, memory loss issues). It invites everyone to find out more about detoxification, supplementation, and more, and guarantees to help you clean up, reduce excess fat, and strengthen your own body.

Part Two: The MS Journey is an invitation to those of you with MS or a similar chronic illness to take charge and impact your wellness. It's important to note that many of the problems associated with MS are also associated with other chronic illnesses such as chronic fatigue syndrome (myalgic encephalomyelitis), fibromyalgia and auto-immune illnesses such as lupus, rheumatoid arthritis, psoriasis, Crohn's disease, ulcerative colitis, type 1 diabetes, and perhaps even glaucoma. Neurologic concerns such as muscle spasms, walking difficulties, and bowel and bladder difficulties are also included in Part Two, and so it is worthwhile to read the book cover to cover no matter who you are.

Getting Started

Following are guidelines to help you get started in a practical and proactive way. Everyone is invited to read Part One. Not all of the suggestions will speak directly to you, but pick and choose those that make sense and begin implementing them in your life right now.

While you are ultimately in charge of how you want to use this book for your best interests, we'd like to offer three suggestions for ways to begin. Don't worry—you don't need to read the book in linear order!

- If you are in a hurry to take action, go directly to Chapter 8: A Few of Our Favorite Things, followed by Dr. Bill's Top 10 Supplement Choices for Reversing Aging, Reducing Pain, and Improving Energy and Brain Function. Circle the items that resonate with you and integrate the ideas and products into your life right now.

- If you have MS or another chronic illness, we suggest you read the entire book, but you may wish to begin with Chapter 9: Dr. Bill's MS Journey: The Beginning and Chapter 10: Dr. Bill's Healthy Discoveries/ Food Sensitivities. You'll get an opportunity to meet Dr. Bill up close and personal. Read through the rest of Part Two and then go back to Part One to round out your education.

- If you have any fatigue, aches and pains, cognitive problems, or chronic pain, read Part One thoroughly and then skim Part Two. But make sure you read Chapter 10: Dr. Bill's Healthy Discoveries/Food Sensitivities, because this is an issue that touches just about everyone.

Remember, no matter how you use this book, you are being proactive in optimizing your health and recovery. Choose those ideas, solutions, and products that make sense to you. Not all suggestions will apply or work for you, but we know most will be helpful, and some will help you a great deal.

Note: We wrote this book together, but you will read Part Two as Dr. Bill writing from the first person. His personal voice will guide you "firsthand" as he takes you through his MS journey and beyond.

PART ONE

The Road to Recovery

*An invitation for everyone with
chronic pain, chronic illness, MS, and auto-immune
disease to take charge and impact your wellness.*

The Road to Recovery

Long-term pain serves no useful function. Chronic pain means recurring, life-disabling intermittent or continuous pain of more than three months' duration. Why three months? Three months means the pain has been present often and recurrent messages are being perceived by the brain that "wind-up" has occurred. Wind-up is a term denoting that the pain has now burned or consistently created a pathway from skin to brain, that it continues to send pain messages even though pain stimulus is gone or complete with scarring. Almost always, chronic pain is called "neuropathic pain," which means "unhappy change" (pathic) "in the nerve or nerves" (neuro). Chronic pain typically indicates that wind-up has occurred.

Neuropathic pain could be thought of best as "irritable" nerve cells that spontaneously fire or are triggered by the tiniest stimulus. A good example is "trigeminal neuralgia," where light touch or even a breeze on that side of the face can trigger a fiery, burning, knife-like pain that can virtually bring a person to his or her knees. As an aside, up to 20% of folks with trigeminal neuralgia will eventually be diagnosed with MS.

Another example of wind-up is a wrist or ankle fracture that becomes recurring, even crippling, pain called RSD, or reflex sympathetic dystrophy. Here, the response of long-term pain after wind-up has occurred is dramatic. Typically it means the skin surface has become shiny, even reddened, and even the bone is less dense on x-ray. Treatment, by freezing the limb with local anesthetic three times in the first three months, is quite effective and may completely solve it. However, if after three months the pain is not gone, it may persist for life and even "spread" to other joint areas. What started as a simple sprain or fracture can become a disabling illness, and no one, not even physicians, can tell when or why this could happen to a person.

Chronic pain afflicts up to 20-30% of Americans today. The pain of arthritis alone troubles 46 million people in the United States. Economic costs, partly healthcare but more so employment, are about $86 billion per year. Traditional medicine's best responses for severe cases are prednisone, NSAIDs (non-steroidal anti-inflammatory drugs) such as ibuprofen and naproxen, and COX-2 inhibitors such as celoxicob (Cele-brex). All of these drugs have potentially very bad side effects, including hip joint death, osteoporosis, bleeding stomach or intestines, injured liver and kidney, and may even cause stroke. Looking at the risk-benefit ratio, we are further amazed to learn that each of the above group of drugs slows down and actually prevents healing. Yes, that NSAID or COX-2 inhibitor you take daily, for relief, can speed up considerably the need for hip or knee replacement!

When Dr. Bill was involved in clinical research on reducing postopera-tive pain after tubal ligation and knee arthroscopy, he co-published articles on this subject. One such article was "Balanced Anesthesia: Why Not Balanced Analgesia?" "Balanced analgesia" means using several drugs to decrease the amount, and hence the side effects, of each drug, resulting in a happier, potentially safer patient. Once again, this happens by balancing the risk-benefit ratio. Here is an explanation of how to balance analgesia (for pain relief) versus balanced anesthesia (for a surgical procedure) with the analogy of balanced diet. The KISS (Keep It Simple Sweetheart) is best followed for ease in learning and teaching.

When we eat a daily balanced diet, we aim to have about 50% of our calories from carbohydrates, preferably unprocessed, 30% from fat, and 20% from protein. To optimize health, it is important to stress fruits, vege-tables, and nuts and to avoid most fast foods, processed foods, and trans fats. Our risk-benefit ratio consideration has us eating as many fresh, natural, locally produced, and whole foods as possible. This minimizes risk from herbicides, pesticides, and preservatives. At the same time, it enhances the benefits from whole nuts, fruits, and vegetables, as they provide more phytonutrients (mini-vitamins), antioxidants, and healthy carbohydrates and fats. Similarly, this variety optimizes health by providing a broad palette of nutrients, so even though people have slightly different genetic make-up they can still reach optimal health. The multivitamin/multi-mineral we suggest fills in potential gaps in nutrients due to the long-term cropping of most of our food sources.

With this illustration of a balanced diet and risk-benefit ratio, we hope to help you appreciate the "balanced anesthesia" your anesthesiologist provides you for a major operation. His or her palette of drugs aim to fine-tune—for your individual physiology, age, and surgical procedure—and allow you to have a safe, relaxed surgery, free from unpleasant memories and with minimal or no pain upon awakening. The anesthesiologist's goal is the three A's: analgesic (pain relief), amnesia (controlled memory loss), and autonomic control (i.e., homeostasis—no wide swings in blood pressure, heart rate, or temperature). To achieve this, in conjunction with optimal operating conditions for your surgeon, they use 1) analgesics (opiates/narcotics, alpha-2 agonists, NSAIDs, nitrous oxide), 2) amnestics (gas or volatile anesthetics, barbiturates, propofol, and benzodiazepines), 3) autonomic control (beta-blockers, calcium channel blockers, alpha-2 agonists, atropine (belladonna), and so on). Finally, to assist the surgeon, muscle relaxants are added to the mix. If local anesthetics are used (spinal, epidural, nerve blocks, or "freezing" agents), all muscle relaxants, analgesics, amnestics, and autonomic control drugs can be minimized. This then permits balanced anesthesia by the anesthesiologists with the best risk-benefit ratio of drugs for the individual patient's physiology. Balanced analgesia preoperatively and postoperatively from a drug risk-benefit ratio includes local anesthetics, narcotics, alpha-2 agonists (e.g., clonidine), NSAIDs (e.g., naproxen, ibuprofen, or ketorolac). We recommend a series of food and food supplements to empower you to control your chronic pain, whatever the source.

Foods and food supplements also have a lot of power, but the changes they bring take a little longer, with side effects that approach zero. This, of course, reduces the risk to you and allows you more flexibility as well as more time to proceed. Subsequent chapters will describe a number of foods and supplements, which together give you some control over your chronic pain. When folks fret about it taking too long, we like to reply, "One thing you do have with chronic pain or illness is time. This enables you to try different and multiple food techniques and choices to determine what works best for you." Side effects of food (outside of allergy) are so minimal you can use any or all of our suggestions in the book. You will then have an empowering road map to follow. So, rather than pain controlling your life, begin with the end in mind—you controlling your pain!

CHAPTER ONE

Body Detoxification

Ask yourself these four questions:

1. Do I believe our air quality is as good as it was 50 years ago?

2. Do I believe our water quality is as good as it was 50 years ago?

3. Do I believe our food quality is as good as it was 50 years ago?

4. Do I believe our environment quality is as good as it was 50 years ago?

Most of us would agree that the answer to these questions is a firm "No." On our journey to wellness, we will address the reality around us as well as within us and will provide you with natural, healthy, and affordable solutions and suggestions to help you on your road to recovery. Part One invites all of you, from people dealing with MS and auto-immune disease to chronic pain and illness, to get informed and be proactive about what you can do right now to build more hope and possibility into your lives. In order to provide you with a comprehensive, step-by-step, progressive coverage of this vast subject, we will begin at the cellular level. Then we'll progress through tissues (i.e., lymph drainage) and then organs (i.e., liver, kidneys, lungs, and skin) and finish with systems (i.e., digestive and central nervous).

We can be proactive in what we breathe, drink, and eat and in the locations in which we choose to work and live. We also need to address the reality that all of us have absorbed many toxins and that it is our job to do a body detoxification program. "Detoxification" is a term oft used and oft misquoted. To an anesthesiologist, "detoxification" means the removal of drugs and drug by-products from a cell and from the body. This applies in particular to drugs acting on the brain and spinal cord. Detoxification also applies to toxic components from our environment. These would include such things as herbicides, pesticides, heavy metals, and large numbers of petrochemical or cleaning agents. The key substance in our body for removing almost every drug used in medicine or anesthesiology is glutathione. (See Chapter 4.) Now that we know how to optimize or raise the glutathione in every cell, we are able to do an ongoing, safe, and continuous detoxification. This will only assist those who have an illness that is partly aggravated by sensitivity to substances that injure or affect brain cells. But before we leap ahead, let's focus on a few other basic pieces of the puzzle.

We now know more about exposure to toxins than we used to because, unfortunately, they have become endemic. It is sobering to think that today's teenagers, for the first time in recorded history, may not live as long as their parents. Each coming generation has more and more risk of auto-immune disease, obesity, diabetes mellitus (types 1 and 2), and especially cancer. As our water, air, diet, and environment deteriorate, our illnesses increase. The substances we are exposed to and ingest have profound influences on our health, especially if they worsen oxidative stress. Following are a couple of stories that, though not pretty, make strong points about toxins in your own life.

Take Off Your Shoes

Air quality has become a real danger. We now know that a child living on a busy street is more likely to develop leukemia than a child on a quiet street. The prime cause of the rise in leukemia is acute automobile, truck, and bus exhaust. Residues from exhaust settle on sidewalks, roads, and lawns. This, in turn, is deposited on floors, carpets, and other surfaces that children play on. Youngsters encounter this exhaust both from the air they breathe and through skin contact.

Skin absorption of toxins is an important issue for all of us, but especially for small children. Obviously this involves minimizing children's contact with petrochemical products (not just gas or solvents), including petroleum jelly (white paraffin in U.K.) and cortiscosteroid creams, and finding alternative ways to deal with rashes and the like. Because today's topical cortisones are stronger and these steroids can have significant effects on bone growth plates, we should, whenever possible, use a topical, non-petrochemical product containing emu oil, shea butter, or almond oil mixtures instead. Other simple measures include the removal of shoes at the door and the change to indoor footwear. I believe the Japanese do this best. This alone greatly reduces everyone's toxic load and protects a crawling toddler as well. In addition, we should favor hardwood, tile, or linoleum and stay away from carpets, which have their own toxins.

Mad Hatters for a Reason

Do you remember the Mad Hatter, the whacky partner of the March Hare who carried on at a tea party in Lewis Carroll's wonderful book *Alice in Wonderland*? The terms "mad as a hatter" and "mad as a March hare" were in common usage for thirty years. The truth is that hat makers, or "hatters," really did go mad. The reason is quite interesting. The most popular hat in the mid-1800s was beaver, but rabbit hats were cheaper. To toughen rabbit-fur fibers, hatters applied a brush solution of mercurous nitrate. Felt made from the shaved fibers was immersed in a boiling acid solution to thicken and harden it. Unfortunately, the acid treatment decomposed the mercurous nitrate to elemental mercury, which was then breathed in and/or swallowed by the hatters. Recurrent exposure to the mercury vapors caused mercury poisoning. Victims developed severe and uncontrollable muscle tremors and twitching limbs, called "hatters' shakes." Secondary troubles included distorted vision and confused speech. Severe cases developed hallucinations and even psychosis. Despite these serious side effects, the use of mercury continued in this way in North America until 1941.

This story can teach us a solid lesson about the use of mercury today. We believe that the removal of dental amalgams may aid in the recovery from many illnesses. Other options to mercury now exist. If your dental practitioner does not believe mercury fillings can cause problems, perhaps you need to change your dental practitioner! Naturally, we appreciate that there are two sides to this discussion, but, due to our neurologic illness, those of us with MS and other such illnesses have more reason than others for anxiety about mercury. Dr. Bill debated whether he should have his mercury amalgams removed. He then met a bright, well-read, just-retired dentist who had taught at three dental schools in Canada and the U.S. and asked the dentist for advice on this matter. The doctor said he would most certainly have the fillings removed, and Dr. Bill followed his counsel.

Dilute, Dilute, Dilute

So what can we do, starting today, to reduce this ever-increasing toxic load? Dilute! Dilution is the solution to pollution. For starters, we need to increase our water intake—not pop, juice, coffee, tea, or alcohol—*water*. Aim for 8-12 glasses per day. Use reverse osmosis to "clean up" tap water or buy bottled water from an ethically researched and documented company. Beware: Up to one-half of most bottled water is simply from the tap! Ozonated spring water should contain no lead, mercury, herbicide, pesticide, or petrochemical contamination. To clean tap water, dechlorinate it using reverse osmosis, a carbon filter, or at least a filtering pitcher, or leave the water standing overnight before drinking it, to allow the chlorine to evaporate out. (If it works for exotic fish, it may help you, too!) It has been reported that over 60,000 chemicals have been found in our water supply. Over the course of a lifetime, we will ingest about 450 pounds of sediment and metals from our drinking water. We hope these statistics will encourage you to seek out purified drinking water.

Secondly, if you need coffee or tea to survive, go organic and prepare them with purified water. Why? Because more weed and insect sprays are used in growing coffee and tea plants than any other agricultural product. Ingesting the coffee or tea means ingesting the deadly sprays too. If you are uncertain and need reinforcement to believe that "we are what we eat," watch the documentary film *Super Size Me*. This movie has had more impact on the fast-food industry than anything else to date. One major hamburger firm is already discontinuing the "super size" policy completely.

Thirdly, pay attention to and minimize your "empty," quick sugar calories. Reduce all pop and all juice cocktails, beverages, and punches—these are primarily fructose, sucrose, and water. Look for juices made from 100% fruit juice. Stay away from artificial sweeteners. If you have a major sweet tooth, learn about stevia, a natural sweetener. Marketing companies have become very skillful in their advertising and can seduce you into purchasing food products that not only have little nutritive value, but also are actually detrimental to your health. Cigarette and alcohol companies have long understood these marketing principles.

You will soon discover that one part of cleaning up our bodies can be done easily—simply by changing what we put into it. Refusing mercury amalgam dental fillings, or having old amalgam removed, will gradually decrease your toxic input. Similarly, by moving to an area with pristine air, clean water, and good soil, you can realize great benefits immediately. Not all of these choices are necessarily affordable, of course, but do what you can; it will not only gradually make a difference, but it will also strengthen your sense of being in control.

Eat Fresh, Eat Fiber

We have found that our parents' generation (people born up until 1945) ate the freshest, best prepared whole foods. This is not because they had more income, but because they had better eating habits and because many had retained the practice of having a vegetable garden. Today, many of us can improve our own habits with the help of community kitchens, food co-ops, and private gardens. Alternatively, it is a great idea to develop a relationship with a farmer/farmers you trust and respect. "Closer to home" eating means more variety (seasonal), fresher produce, and more control over how your food is grown.

What would be another method of cleaning up our bodies? More fiber. Soluble and non-soluble (ground flax contains both) will "scrub" your intestines and help eliminate toxic wastes excreted by the liver into the bile, including the "bad cholesterol," LDL. Cooked legumes and whole grains are other excellent sources of fiber—but not wheat, barley, or rye if you are gluten sensitive (celiac disease). Fresh fruits and vegetables are very good. Consuming wholesome food is, by far, preferable to cleansing regimes that bubble air, ozone, coffee, water, saline, or x-ray dye up our butts, but this is, of course, a personal decision.

WHY MORE FIBER?

- *Carry away toxic wastes*
- *"Scrub" the intestine*
- *Slow absorption of simple sugars into the bloodstream*
- *Reduce work of the liver*
- *Carry away LDL (bad cholesterol)*
- *Reduce constipation*
- *Feed "friendly" bacteria in the colon*

Should juice or water fasts be considered? If you want to go this cleansing route, take some time off. We have a physician cousin who died of a heart attack while he was working hard breaking in horses during a three-day fast. Doing "one thing at a time" will be difficult for the Type-A workaholics out there—some of whom have MS and other chronic diseases.

What supplements can assist this detox and body cleansing approach? Fresh water, fruit and/or vegetable shakes or smoothies, and foods containing plenty of fiber should be among your first choices. "Fiber cookies" are one easy option. The multivitamin/multi-mineral combined with vitamin D, calcium, and magnesium will also contribute to the cleansing process. Boosting our endogenous antioxidant, glutathione (pronounced "glue-the-tie-on"), inside the cell with a very good whey protein isolate, high in bioactive cysteine will have a profoundly beneficial effect. Glutathione is the number one molecule for detoxing or removing almost all drugs, heavy metals (e.g., mercury, lead, and cadmium), petrochemical residues, tobacco-triggered free radicals, tar, and most herbicides and pesticides. Glutathione is, without question, our most optimal and cheapest detoxification ally. Water would be the only exception to this.

Milk and Whey Protein

Many well-respected doctors have documented the health benefits of taking whey protein isolate (bioactive cysteine), an essential building block of our body cells. This product can be found in pouches of fine, white powder (see *Appendix A & B*) made from cow's milk. It is an excellent product for oral chelation, too, and provides building blocks for glutathione, which we will discuss later. In reality, any mammalian milk will have the same effect, and the very best of these, of course, is fresh human breast milk. However, as adults we do not have access to this option!

Those of you who are great fans of the Paleolithic or Stone Age diet will no doubt feel this recommendation is blasphemy for someone with MS. All mammalian milk contains butyrophilin, which is a probable trigger for molecular mimicry, causing our own white blood cells (immune response) to pick on the myelin sheath around our nerves in our brain and spinal cord. However, this particular whey protein isolate, providing bioactive cysteine, is completely defatted and all the casein protein is removed as well. In most but not all cases of milk sensitivity (allergy), the casein (cheese) component is the cause. Only one in 100,000 will be allergic to this very clean whey protein isolate. In addition, 99% of the lactose, the sugar in the milk, is removed. This means that most people should have no problem, except for those who are extremely lactose sensitive. If you are lactose intolerant, take a lactase supplement with the whey or a quality plant digestive enzyme that includes lactase.

More information on the milk sensitivity issue can be found in a research paper by Drs. Toohey, Smith, and Hickey published in April 2000 in the *British Journal of Nutrition*. We had the good fortune of hearing Dr. Lynn Toohey speak on this issue in Vancouver in 2002, where she outlined the three most common triggers of food sensitivity and potential causes of auto-immune diseases such as MS and rheumatoid arthritis. The three common triggers were lectins from wheat, red kidney beans, and casein. In personal discussion with Dr. Toohey later, we found out that the primary problem was from the casein in cow's milk, not the whey.

Infrared Sauna Therapy

Infrared energy is a form of heat energy. Our sun produces most of its energy in the infrared segment of the light spectrum in the 7-14 micron range (a micron is 1/100,000 of a meter). Our bodies radiate infrared energy in the range of 8-14 microns through the skin. Infrared therapy helps detoxify the body through enhancing blood flow and promoting perspiration. Thus there is an alternative method of detoxification that can be used: the infrared sauna. These small (2-4 people) sauna units, for home or shared use, emit radiant heat in the form of infrared energy. This means that radiant heat travels from the source to your body without having to heat the air in between.

In 1965 Dr. Tadashi Ishikawa, of Fuji Medical Research and Development, received a patent for a zirconia ceramic infrared heater, but until 1979 only medical practitioners in Japan were able to use these infrared thermal systems. The systems were then released for use worldwide and have been sold in North America since 1981. A common use of infrared heat for many years has been warming newborns and postoperative patients. Our own infrared sauna is made of red cedar from Canada's west coast and is designed with the Japanese technology described here (see *Appendix A & B*).

A conventional sauna relies on an indirect means of heat (convection and conduction) and operates at 180-235 degrees Fahrenheit. Infrared saunas operate at 50-125 degrees Fahrenheit, or 10-60 degrees Celsius, allowing its user to breathe cooler air while still feeling warmth. This is a welcomed relief for the "cold, cold hands and feet" symptom of people with MS.

Over the last 25 years, primarily Japanese and Chinese researchers have completed extensive research on infrared heat treatment. Their findings support infrared therapy as a method of healing. Over 700,000 infrared thermal systems have been sold in the Orient alone, and some 30 million people have received localized infrared treatment worldwide. In Germany, physicians have used whole-body infrared therapy for over 80 years. The widespread use of infrared heat and its consequent acceptance by Health Canada and the FDA in the United States strongly suggests that it is safe.

Now that we have established safety, what might infrared sauna therapy do for those of us who have chronic illnesses, especially MS? One benefit for MS folks using infrared heat to produce cardiovascular conditioning. "Regular use of a sauna may impart a similar stress on the cardiovascular system as running or jogging, and its regular use may be as effective a means of cardiovascular conditioning and burning of calories as regular exercise."[1]

WHY INFRARED SAUNA?

- *Increased blood flow to help healing*
- *Increased burning of energy (calories) by the body*
- *Increased cardiac workout*
- *Speeds toxin removal from fat cells*
- *Release of toxins via perspiration*

No doubt you may be wondering, "What if my MS and I cannot tolerate heat?" If this is the case, you should move forward slowly and gradually with time and patience. An infrared sauna makes it possible for people in wheelchairs and those who cannot follow an exercise/conditioning program to achieve a cardiovascular training effect. Initially, you can leave the sauna door open. This minimizes the ambient heat while allowing the infrared to still penetrate and do most of its good. We now know that heat worsens symptoms of most central nervous system (CNS) illnesses, including stroke and MS. However, most symptoms subside once cooling to normal temperature occurs.

---

[1] *Journal of the American Medical Association* (7 August 1981).

In addition, nerves that have lost their myelin are particularly sensitive to heat—that would apply to MS! This may explain why 70% of MS patients are very heat sensitive. I was but, happily, am less so now.

Why, then, would we consider infrared therapy? It ties in, in three ways. First, the improved blood flow stimulates healing in all parts of the body, including our skin, brain, and spinal cord. Second, the caloric consumption controls weight gain. Guyton's *Text of Medical Physiology* states that one gram of sweat uses 0.586 calories. The *Journal of the American Medical Association* goes on to state, "A moderately conditioned person can easily sweat off 500 grams in a sauna, consuming nearly 300 calories—the equivalent of running two to three miles. A heat-conditioned person can easily sweat off 600-800 calories with no adverse effects. While the weight of water loss can be regained by rehydration, the calories consumed will not be."[2] Hence, the infrared sauna can help us with both weight control and cardiovascular conditioning. Third, detoxification is accomplished through sweating (perspiration). The infrared heat penetrates 3-4 centimeters (1.5-2 inches) beneath our skin. Our fat layer is usually here and the increased circulation caused by the infrared will help the whole body to detoxify. When using a sauna, remember to replace your minerals too, especially sodium and potassium. And drink lots of water!

In summary, detoxification is achieved in many different ways. It is up to each of us to work out the option that is best and most affordable to us. If you do not handle heat well, you must start slowly and carefully and should not think about making a sauna purchase before being totally comfortable with it. Exercise, discussed in Chapter 15 on movement, is also a superb way to detoxify through sweating. Again, with exercise you must begin slowly and build up a tolerance. Careful detoxification with the whey protein isolate is an option for almost everyone. And, as mentioned, ample water intake is a must. Remember, "Dilution is the secret to pollution!"

---

[2] Ibid.

CHAPTER TWO

Supplementation for Optimal Health

Nutritional supplementation has become a burgeoning industry. Why? We believe it is because people's mindsets have shifted. Many people, especially the well informed, are now aiming for optimal health. In fact, it is now felt that 75-80% of our chronic health problems are nutrition based. In this chapter, we outline three food pyramids to demonstrate how we as a culture should be changing our emphasis from disease to wellness. Then we present why vitamin/mineral supplements are needed and provide

It is now felt that 75-80% of our chronic health problems are nutrition based.

tips on choosing supplements. Finally, we take a brief look at the role vitamins and minerals play in the body, the amounts recommended by the government, and our recommendations for chronic illness and optimal health.

Food Pyramids Point the Way

In January 2005, new dietary guidelines for Americans were released, which were later depicted in a new food pyramid. The new guidelines place a greater emphasis on reducing caloric intake for weight control and increasing physical activity (60-90 minutes daily). In addition, people are encouraged to get all of their nutrients solely from food. The new guidelines also recognize that certain population groups need vitamin supplements. These include vitamin B-12 for people over 50 and supplemental vitamin D for dark-skinned people as well as the elderly.

MyPyramid (Figure 1), from the United States Department of Agriculture, translates dietary guidelines into recommended food intake. MyPyramid is the newest food pyramid for Americans. It provides a personalized approach to healthy eating and physical activity; all you need to do is key in your age and sex on its website. It features the following food groups: Grains, Vegetables, Fruits, Oils, Milk, and Meat & Beans, and specifies food choices that will improve the typical diet. Using MyPyramid will help you increase your intake of vitamins, minerals, and dietary fiber as well as lower your intake of saturated fats, trans fats, and cholesterol. The recommended calorie intake is balanced against physical activity to prevent weight gain and/or to promote a healthy weight.

MyPyramid has several advantages. It points consumers in the direction of healthy eating and comes with colorful graphics and a wealth of information that can be accessed at the click of a mouse. This includes food selection, food preparation, portion sizes, menus, nutrients in each food group and their health benefits, as well as guidance on physical activity.

MyPyramid also has disadvantages. We feel that, in some respects, the pyramid does not go far enough in its recommendations. The guidelines for grains are to make half of your servings whole grain. We feel that all servings of grains should be whole grains. Processed grains should be reserved for special occasions only. The recommendations for oils should emphasize a daily intake of omega-3 fats and should discourage the intake of any trans fats.

Because the pyramid is for healthy people, it would not be complete enough for someone suffering from a chronic illness or health condition. A consultation with a dietician or nutrition specialist would be necessary to adjust your food intake to meet your individual needs. Because access to the pyramid information is via the internet, it requires the use of a computer as well as reading skills. Lastly, the pyramid is based on a food intake that would meet the Recommended Daily Allowance (RDA) for vitamins, minerals, and other nutrients. It does not take into consideration the amounts of nutrients we need to go beyond general health into the realm of disease prevention and optimal health.

A food guide is also available in Canada. Canada's Food Guide to Healthy Eating is represented by a rainbow, with the colored arcs of the rainbow featuring food groups. Its concepts are similar to MyPyramid, but it does not have the individualization made possible by computer. A new food guide is due to be released in Canada within the next year.

The "Mediterranean" Food Pyramid (Figure 1) is from a cultural group that suffers less heart disease than we have in North America. The greatest difference here is the emphasis on olive oil, a monounsaturated fatty acid.

The third and perhaps ultimate pyramid is the "Optimal Nutrition" Food Pyramid designed by Dr. Roy Walford in his book *Beyond the 120 Year Diet*. Dr. Walford has shifted fruits, vegetables, beans, and nuts to the anchor or dominant position, meaning the diet should emphasize these foods. Carbohydrates are assigned a position on the glycemic index (GI), which ranks them on their ability to raise blood sugar levels. The lower the rating, the slower the body converts the food to blood sugar. For example, boiled potato, which is easy for the body to digest and convert to blood sugar, has a glycemic index of 88. Chickpeas, on the other hand, because of their fiber and other nutrients, take longer for body to convert to glucose (blood sugar) and therefore have a lower glycemic index—28. Foods that are low in *complex* carbohydrates and high in *simple* carbohydrates, such as cornflakes and sweet donuts, would be assigned a high GI. Foods such as broccoli, apples, "grainy" whole wheat bread, and brown rice would be assigned a low GI.

One concern with high GI foods is their ability to cause a rapid and high increase in insulin in the blood. This is the body's way of lowering blood sugar. However, blood sugar levels may then come crashing down

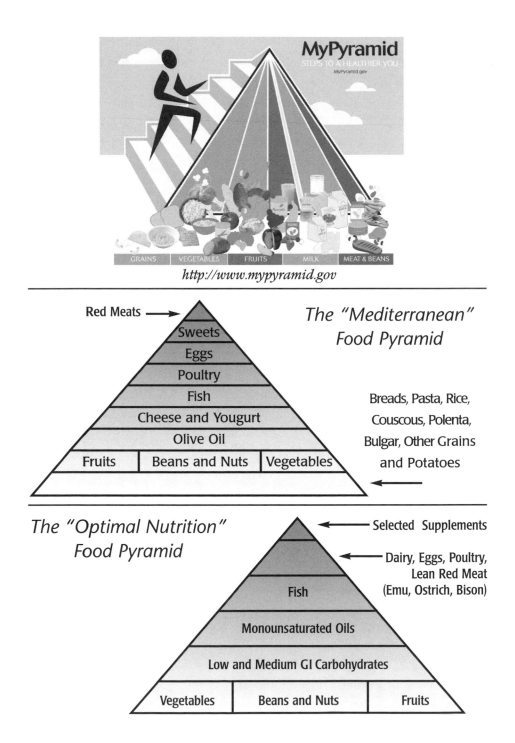

http://www.mypyramid.gov

too low, triggering a feeling of hunger and leading to overeating. In some people, especially when weight is a problem, the body develops insulin resistance, and blood sugar and insulin levels remain high. The blood sugar is then directed into fat stores. You should eat foods with a low glycemic index so that 1) your blood glucose is controlled, 2) your cholesterol level is controlled, and 3) your appetite is controlled. This, in turn, will lower your risk of heart disease and type 2 diabetes.

The vast majority of carbohydrates consumed should be in the low to medium GI range. Avoid simple sugars and refined foods. Instead, reach for vegetables with your meals. Choose unprocessed whole grains, whole-grain products, and lentils whenever you can. Remember, though, that using the glycemic index to choose foods is only one strategy for healthy eating. In his food pyramid, Dr. Walford also puts selected supplements at the top. He recognizes that many or most of us are unable to obtain all of our body's needs from the food that is readily available to us. We agree with him and believe that everyone should eat according to his food pyramid as well as take vitamin, mineral, and other supplements regularly. As a final note, it takes five to six times as much nutrition to *reverse* a condition that's already in place as it does to *prevent* problems.

Our Diets Have Changed

Genetically, humans are "old" beings, as we probably haven't changed for hundreds of thousands of years. Our diet, by comparison, has changed drastically in just the last 10,000 years with the agricultural revolution, the discovery of fire, and our habitation now spanning the majority of the earth's surface. All of these changes have an impact on our dietary requirements and on what our dietary intakes should be. It is thought that 10,000 years ago, over the course of a year, we ate some 200 different seeds, nuts, fruits, and other foods. Today, we would be hard pressed to name more than 20 major foods in our diets. Most of these are based on wheat, rice, soy, corn, milk products, and a number of common vegetables—especially in North America—such as peas, beans, carrots, and corn. Further limiting our variety is our ability to get most foods all year long by importing them from elsewhere. This often results in our eating a single variety of fruit or vegetable (for instance, only iceberg lettuce or Granny Smith apples).

All of these factors have made a difference. One other difference in our modern lifestyle is that we have moved to more temperate climates—that is, further away from the equator. This has had an impact on us as well, because most of us now live in areas where we can't make much vitamin D from the sun.

Since 2000, two very amazing developments have occurred with respect to nutrition recommendations. First, more traditional organizations began to recommend vitamin/mineral supplementation. In 2000 and again in 2005, the United States Department of Agriculture (USDA) Dietary Guidelines for Americans recognized that some people need a vitamin/mineral supplement to meet specific nutrient needs. The American Dietetic Association (ADA) has also adopted a policy statement addressing the use of nutritional supplements for some individuals. We applaud the American Medical Association (AMA), who published in their journal in 2002 that most Americans would benefit from a daily multivitamin/multi-mineral supplement. Many nutrition researchers, scientists, and health professionals have been advocating vitamin/mineral supplements and other dietary supplements for quite some time. As science continues to shed light on the roles of nutrients and the optimum amounts and combinations for health and for disease prevention, recommendations for dietary supplementation will continue to evolve.

The second development was the July 2002 *Scientific American* article by Walter C. Willett and Meir J. Stampfer, professors of epidemiology and nutrition at the Harvard School of Public Health and professors of medicine at Harvard Medical School. They set out to improve upon the USDA Food Pyramid. Their "New Food Pyramid" is even more forward thinking than Walford's pyramid. In the New Food Pyramid, Willett and Stampfer distinguish between healthy and unhealthy fats and carbohydrates. Healthy fats include liquid vegetable oils such as olive, canola, soy, corn, sunflower, and peanut. Trans fat does not appear in the pyramid. Healthy carbohydrates include whole grain foods such as oatmeal and brown rice. Willett and Stampfer recommend avoiding refined carbohydrates, butter, and red meat. The New Food Pyramid features multivitamins for most, and alcohol in moderation. In addition, it includes *daily* exercise (walking or running) as the base of the pyramid. The New Food Pyramid represents advanced thinking. Unfortunately, not everyone, including healthcare professionals, has accepted these wise changes.

No matter how well we eat, it is increasingly difficult to get all of the nutrition we need from food alone.

We certainly advocate a diet based on whole foods, fresh foods, and natural foods, preferably organic. We advise reducing the consumption of processed, packaged, and commercial foods, as this will help you avoid excess salt, sugar, and trans fat, all of which are known to have a negative impact on health. In addition, these foods usually have higher levels of additives and preservatives. They often provide fewer nutrients and more calories. However, as mentioned, no matter how well we eat, it is increasingly difficult to get all of the nutrition we need from food alone.

Why Supplement?

The following reasons illustrate the need for vitamins, minerals, and other dietary supplements:

1. Crop nutrient losses: Our soils are becoming depleted of minerals, leading to a reduced mineral content in many crops. According to one study, six minerals have been reduced by as much as 76% in the last 50 years. Another study by the University of Texas in 2004 reported a 38% decline in riboflavin (B vitamin) and a 20% decline in vitamin C as well as decreases in protein, calcium, and phosphorus in 43 common garden crops.

2. Poor digestion is common among the elderly. Reduced gastric juices, lack of friendly gut bacteria, and stress can all impair digestion, making it more difficult to assimilate the nutrients in food.

3. Microwave cooking alters the nutrition provided by a food.

4. Storage can reduce the nutritional value of food, especially fruits and vegetables. The average distance food travels from field to table can be as much as 2,000 miles.

5. Food restriction because of weight loss diets, food allergies, or food avoidance can result in poor nutritional intakes.

6. Poor lifestyle habits such as smoking, drinking alcohol, and consuming caffeine can replace important foods, interfere with the absorption of nutrients, or lead to nutrient loss from the body.

7. Stress, either physical or emotional, increases the body's need for vitamins, minerals, and other nutrients.

8. Nutrient imbalances can impair how the body uses nutrients. No single nutrient can do the job alone. The body relies on a network of nutrients to stay healthy. Therefore, a balance of nutrients is needed.

9. Variances exist in the nutrient content of foods.

10. Food selection can have an impact on the nutritional value of a person's diet. If only a few different foods are regularly eaten, then the types and amounts of vitamins, minerals, and other valuable nutrients will be low.

National surveys indicate that about half of the population in North America uses supplements. Those who do tend to be healthy and have positive attitudes about their diets and health. Surveys have shown that the use of supplements among healthcare professionals (including physicians, dieticians, and pharmacists) is high. People who use supplements often have healthy diets as well as healthy lifestyle habits, such as exercising and not smoking. Supplements *should not* be an excuse to eat poorly, skip exercise, and neglect other healthy habits. Rather, supplements can be a form of "health insurance" toward good health. A healthy diet supplies thousands of other vital components needed for health, such as fiber, essential fats, minerals, antioxidants, and phytonutrients (biologically active compounds).

How to Choose?

Choosing a supplement can be difficult. The supplement market is a billion-dollar industry with hundreds of companies producing a confusing array of bottles and potions. How to choose? First of all, a multivitamin with minerals should provide 100% of the Daily Value for all or most vitamins and a number of minerals. Most vitamin/mineral supplements will not be able to provide the full RDA of calcium. This is because calcium is needed in a large amount and is a bulky nutrient. Some calcium may need to be taken separately. A multivitamin with minerals can fill nutrient gaps, protect health, and reduce the risk of disease.

Supplements should not be an excuse to eat poorly, skip exercise, and neglect other healthy habits. Rather, supplements can be a form of "health insurance" toward good health.

How to Judge Quality?

Now that you have an overview of supplements, what are the criteria for judging among the several hundred thousand brands of vitamin/mineral supplements? One option you have as a consumer is to call the manufacturer directly. Some questions to ask are:

- Does the company have its own research scientists?
- Does the company own farms that grow plants?
- Does the company do its own testing for quality, strength, and purity?
- Does the company do clinical trials on its products?

A "yes" to these questions indicates a good nutrition company. Another option is to consult nutrition experts who have had experience with a variety of products. They will know which ones have a proven track record and which ones are perhaps not so good. Also, try to determine that the supplement:

- Uses exclusively natural vitamin E containing a mixture of tocopherols.

- Uses optimum amounts of antioxidants: 200-400 IU vitamin E, 200-500 mg vitamin C, 5,000-15,000 IU beta-carotene, and 70-200 mcg selenium. Limits vitamin A acetate or palmitate to no more than 4,000 IU.

- Uses optimum amounts of bone nutrients: 500-1,500 mg calcium, 210-700 mg magnesium, 200-800 IU vitamin D, and at least 1 mg boron (40 mcg vitamin K allowed in the United States, but not in Canada).

- Uses optimum amounts of B vitamins involved to lower homocysteine levels and reduce heart disease: at least 400 mcg folic acid, 1.7 mg vitamin B-6, and 6 mcg vitamin B-12.

- Provides significant amounts of carotenoids such as lutein and lycopene.

- Provides significant amounts of flavonoids from many sources (e.g., quercetin, isoflavones, grape seed extract).

- Uses well-absorbed, bioavailable sources of trace minerals (e.g., chromium, copper, manganese, iron, zinc, etc). Check to see that the minerals are chelated. (Chelated minerals are bound to protein and easier for the body to absorb.) To check for chelation, look for the following on the label: zinc as zinc chelate; magnesium as magnesium chelate, and so on.

- Capsules should dissolve within 30 minutes; coated tablets should dissolve within 45 minutes. The supplement should have the USP designation on the label, meaning that the supplement meets standards for disintegration (how it breaks into small pieces), dissolution (how it dissolves), strength, and purity.

- The product's bottle should show an expiration date.

For best results with supplements, keep the following in mind:

- Take supplements with meals. The food will help the body absorb the vitamins and minerals.

- Take supplements as directed on the bottle. More is *not* better.

- Avoid taking supplements with coffee, tea, or sodas. These beverages can interfere with the absorption of the minerals.

- Take a balanced supplement. The nutrients work together. For example, calcium needs magnesium for best results in the body.

- If you have trouble swallowing supplements, first place a small amount of liquid in your mouth, then pop in the capsules. Follow with a good gulp of liquid. Some people find that liquids thicker than water work better for swallowing capsules. Or, you might want to use a liquid with lots of flavour, such as orange or grape juice. If swallowing any tablet or capsule is a crisis, dissolve them in a liquid or use liquid products.

Our bodies need many different nutrients. First and foremost, you need to eat a healthy diet. This would be a diet rich in fruits, vegetables, whole grains, legumes, nuts, seeds, and lean protein. Organic foods have frequently been shown to be higher in essential nutrients than conventionally grown foods. Our bodies need more than 50 essential nutrients from vitamins, minerals, proteins, fats, and carbohydrates. Eating a variety of foods will help ensure that you get these nutrients. In addition, foods contain other nutrients that are vital to our health and longevity. For example, plants contain over 12,000 phytonutrients that help the plant to grow well and ward off diseases and pests. When we eat plants, the benefits of the phytonutrients are passed on to us. Remember, though, that moderate portion sizes of all foods are important to prevent weight gain.

To help you better understand why we need a variety of nutrients, we have taken the major vitamins and minerals and grouped them as follows:

1. Bone-Related Nutrients: calcium, phosphorus, magnesium, vitamin D, fluoride, vitamin K, and boron.

2. The B Vitamins: vitamins B-1, B-2, B-3, B-6, folic acid, B-12, pantothenic acid, and biotin.

3. Additional Vitamins and Trace Minerals: vitamin A, carotenoids, chromium, copper, iodine, iron, manganese, molybdenum, and zinc.

4. The Antioxidants: vitamin C, vitamin E, selenium, alpha-lipoic acid, Coenzyme Q-10, and glutathione.

For each group, we have outlined information on the role of the nutrient in the body, the food sources that contain it, and recommendations for supplements. At the end of the section, you will find a handy chart with recommendations for daily intake of each nutrient as well as for supplementation. To best find the information you need, we suggest you either:

- Read the entire section

- Skip to the nutrients that interest you

- Or, if you just want to know how much you should have for a certain nutrient, turn to the chart on pages 41-46.

1. Bone-Related Nutrients

The main nutrients needed for healthy bones include calcium, phosphorus, magnesium, vitamin D, fluoride, boron, and vitamin K. Dr. Bill is especially interested in these nutrients as he is quite at risk for osteoporosis, which refers to thin, fragile bones. His mom has lost four inches in height and her ribs ride on her pelvis. Dr. Bill has osteopenia (mild osteoporosis) of his legs and osteoporosis in his spine.

Calcium:

Besides building bones and teeth, calcium plays a role in nerve transmission, muscle contraction, and dilation of blood vessels. Over 99% of the body's calcium is in the bones and teeth. Bone undergoes constant breakdown and rebuilding. In aging adults, the rate of breakdown is greater than that of rebuilding. This leads to bones that become fragile and easily broken. Significant bone loss is known as osteoporosis. People with osteoporosis are at great risk of breaking bones and having the bones in the spine collapse. If folks with MS or chronic illness are inactive, their osteoporosis risk is increased. In addition, many people with auto-immune illness or chronic illness are prescribed corticosteroid medications such as Prednisone. Corticosteroids dramatically increase the risk of osteoporosis.

The best food sources of calcium are dairy products, tofu, kale, spinach, broccoli, nuts, canned sardines/salmon with bones, molasses, cooked dried peas, and beans.

Dietary surveys reveal that most adults do not obtain sufficient calcium from food. Therefore, most adults should consider a calcium supplement of 500-1,000 mg/day. When choosing a supplement, look for the amount of *elemental* calcium as written on the label. Aim to take calcium carbonate supplements with meals to improve absorption. Other forms of calcium supplements do not need to be taken with food for best absorption. There are many different forms of calcium supplements on the market. They come as liquid, chewables, tablets, and capsules. Avoid bone meal and dolomite calcium supplements as they may contain lead. Remember, for best absorption, take your calcium supplement in doses of 500 mg or less. When taken in larger doses, less of the calcium is absorbed.

Phosphorus:

Phosphorus has many roles in the body. Like calcium, most of the phosphorus in the body is in the bones and teeth. Because phosphorus is widely distributed in foods, deficiency is extremely rare.

Magnesium:

Magnesium is involved in over 300 enzyme systems in the body and is needed for energy production. Over half of the magnesium in our bodies is in the bones. Magnesium intake can be low, especially in people who rely on processed foods. Best sources of magnesium are tofu, legumes, seeds, nuts, whole grains, and leafy green vegetables.

Vitamin D:

Vitamin D is needed for absorption of calcium and for building bones and teeth. While the best source of vitamin D is the sun's rays, food sources are extremely limited. People living at more northern latitudes such as the northern United States and Canada cannot make vitamin D in their bodies year-round. This, and the limited amount of vitamin D in food, makes these people at high risk of vitamin D deficiency.

Best food sources of vitamin D include fluid milk and fortified soy and rice drinks. Butter and eggs contain small amounts of vitamin D. Vitamin D is also added to margarines. The richest natural source of vitamin D is fish, especially fish liver oil. However, do not attempt to meet your vitamin D needs with fish liver oil. Fish liver oil is very high in vitamin A, and taking extra fish liver oil to boost vitamin D intake can result in a toxic intake of vitamin A.

Vitamin D supplements given to people during the winter months have been documented to improve mood. Historically, our bodies were programmed to make vitamin D from exposure to sunshine. Now, we live more of an "indoor" existence with limited exposure to the sun. In addition, people use sunscreen and clothing to block the sun's rays on their skin. The consequence is that less vitamin D is produced in the skin. Furthermore, as we age, we produce about one-fourth the vitamin D compared to when we were younger. Dark-skinned people are at a greater disadvantage. They require two hours or more in the sun to produce the same amount of vitamin D that a light-skinned person produces in 20 minutes.

We feel that the current recommendations for vitamin D are too low. Vitamin D plays a critical role in bone health, in prevention of cancer, in prevention of auto-immune disease, and in influencing mood. Indeed, Dr. Bill feels that vitamin D has played a critical role in improving his MS and depression. Vitamin D is perhaps more of a hormone in its action in the body than a vitamin. There is ample evidence from Dr. Reinhold Vieth's work in Canada and from other researchers that higher levels of vitamin D are required and that up to 4,000 IU/day is safe. See Chapter 5 on vitamin D for details.

Fluoride:

Fluoride helps to stimulate the formation of bones and teeth. It also protects against dental caries.

Vitamin K:

Vitamin K is important for healthy bones. It is also needed in the production of at least 4 of the 13 proteins involved in blood clotting. A deficiency of vitamin K results in slow blood clotting and, in severe cases, bleeding. Vitamin K is found in dark-green leafy vegetables, such as Brussels sprouts, lettuce, broccoli, spinach, and kale. It is also found in liver, egg yolks, herbal tea, and green tea. Some vitamin K is also produced by the beneficial bacteria in our large bowel.

Vitamin K is not sold in supplements in Canada. The reason is that vitamin K interacts with the drug warfarin (Coumadin), which is used to thin the blood in order to prevent clotting. Alternatives for those folks unable to tolerate warfarin include heparin (injected under the skin), aspirin (81-325 mg), or plenty of omega-3 oils or fish oils. Omega-3 oils help to prevent blood from clotting.

Boron:

Boron enhances the absorption of calcium magnesium and phosphorus. It also affects the structure and strength of bones. Fruits, vegetables, nuts, and legumes are particularly rich in boron.

2. The B Vitamins

The eight B vitamins are: thiamin (B-1), riboflavin (B-2), niacin (B-3), pantothenic acid (B-5), pyridoxine (B-6), cyanocobalamin (B-12), folic acid, and biotin. All are water soluble and short lived in the body, so toxicity is quite rare.

Thiamin (B-1):

The main function of thiamin is to help convert carbohydrates into energy. Deficiency of thiamin causes loss of energy, nerve damage, and muscular weakness. Chronic alcoholics are at risk of thiamin deficiency. Thiamin also helps to produce acetylcholine, a chemical in the brain that helps with information storage and retrieval. Thiamin activates serotonin, our "feel good" brain chemical. Some studies have shown that taking a 50 mg thiamin supplement results in clearer thinking, more energy, and better sleep.

Among the most important food sources of thiamin are whole grains, pork, liver, and cooked dried beans and peas. Many flour and grain products are fortified with thiamin. Thiamin is sensitive to heat and is easily leached out of the food into the cooking water.

Riboflavin (B-2):

Riboflavin acts with many enzymes to convert food into energy. It is also involved in red blood cell formation, the absorption of iron, the metabolism of B-6, and the production of serotonin and dopamine (neurotransmitters). As with thiamin, recent studies reported that a

50 mg supplement of riboflavin resulted in improved mood and clearer thinking.

Because riboflavin is abundant in the food supply, deficiency is rare. Meats, fish, whole grains, milk products, vegetables, and legumes all contain riboflavin. In addition, riboflavin is added to flour and grain products.

Niacin (B-3):

Like riboflavin and thiamin, niacin helps convert food into energy. Niacin is also needed for making fatty acids and steroids. Furthermore, niacin is involved in DNA replication and repair. Niacin deficiency is known as pellagra and can occur in chronic alcoholism.

Large doses of niacin are sometimes used to treat high blood cholesterol. However, these high doses can cause blood vessels to dilate and result in flushing. To reduce the flushing effect, newer niacin formulations are slow release. High doses of niacin (3-9 g/day) can be toxic to the liver when taken over a prolonged period. Your healthcare practitioner should monitor this if these amounts are being used.

Best food sources are liver, eggs, fish, peanuts, legumes, whole grains, avocadoes, milk, broccoli, pork, potatoes, tomatoes, and wheat germ.

Pyridoxine (B-6):

B-6 plays an important role in protein metabolism, helping to make amino acids and to break them down for conversion into other compounds or energy. This vitamin is needed to synthesize muscle protein, hemoglobin, insulin, and antibodies, which protect against infection. Vitamin B-6 is essential for the brain to produce serotonin from tryptophan, an amino acid. In addition, B-6 is needed to make DHA, a critical fat needed by the brain. Studies show that people with low DHA levels are more likely to be depressed and that B-6 supplements improve the mood of depressed people.

According to some researchers, almost half of all women consume less than half of the RDA for vitamin B-6. In addition, 75% of young women who are restricting calories are deficient in B-6. Other researchers have found that about half of men and women over 50 get the recommended amount of B-6 in their diets. Thus, supplemental B-6 is needed to achieve adequate levels of this vitamin.

Vitamin B-6 is found in a wide variety of foods, including meats, fish, nuts, beans, whole grains, and some fruits and vegetables.

Folate (Folic Acid):

This B vitamin is important for DNA metabolism and cell division and tissue growth. It is also involved in the formation of hemoglobin in red blood cells. Folate is found in green leafy vegetables, peas, oranges, carrots, eggs, bananas, avocado, whole grain, yeast, and liver. Folate is easily lost in cooking and in the processing of foods.

The average intake of folate has been determined to be 242 mcg. It is thought that an additional 100 mcg would be obtained from fortified foods. Thus, many adults do not get enough folate from food, and a folic acid supplement of 400 mcg is therefore recommended. A folic acid supplement is also recommended for all women of child-bearing age, especially in the months before conception. This is because folic acid prevents neural tube birth defects, which occur in the first few weeks of pregnancy. Higher levels of folic acid supplementation (5 mg) are recommended in women who have had a miscarriage or who have had a child born with a neural tube defect. Because of the importance of folic acid in preventing birth defects, many foods are now fortified with folic acid.

There is considerable evidence that folic acid may reduce the risk of heart disease and stroke by reducing homocysteine. Homocysteine is a protein in the blood, and high levels of this protein have been found in people suffering from heart disease and stroke. Normally, homocysteine is recycled through metabolic reactions with the help of folic acid, vitamin B-12, and vitamin B-6. A level of 1,000 ug (1,000 mcg) of folic acid is recommended for people with heart disease. It is not known at this time how much supplemental folic acid would be best for prevention of heart disease or stroke. Levels up to 5 mg are currently being researched. However, keep in mind that the Upper Level of Tolerable Intake is 1,000 mcg. Too much can be a problem, as high amounts of folic acid can cover up symptoms of vitamin B-12 deficiency. Also, there is a concern about people getting too much folate when all sources of folate (food, supplements, and food fortification) are considered.

Over one-third of depressed people are deficient in folic acid, yet the role of folic acid in improving mood has largely been ignored. In a study of depressed older patients, folic acid has been shown to improve mood. The improvement experienced with folate alone was better than that experienced with many antidepressants. Folate does this by helping the body to produce more s-adenosyl methionine or SAMe, a chemical important to mood.

Additionally, evidence exists that folate may prevent Alzheimer's disease and Parkinson's disease. Interestingly, high levels of homocysteine have also been reported in people with these two conditions.

Vitamin B-12:

Like folate, B-12 is needed for DNA metabolism. It is also needed for red blood cell formation and maintenance of the nervous system. Animal foods contain B-12, while no plant foods do. However, certain microorganisms, used to ferment foods, can make some B-12. Soy sauce, miso, and tempeh are fermented foods that may contain B-12.

For certain people, absorption of B-12 from food can be a problem. In order to absorb B-12, people need a substance called intrinsic factor, which is secreted by the stomach. The intrinsic factor separates the B-12 from the protein to which it is attached, making it available for absorption. If a person lacks intrinsic factor, B-12 absorption from food is not possible. In addition, stomach acid is needed to absorb B-12. In some of us, less stomach acid is produced as we age. This can cause malabsorption of B-12, too. Supplemental B-12, either by injection or by capsules, is needed to prevent pernicious anemia. If the anemia is severe, it can be followed by nerve damage.

Because many people over 50 have low stomach acid and therefore may not absorb dietary B-12 very well, it is recommended that they get their B-12 from fortified foods or supplements. All elderly or neurologically challenged individuals should supplement B-12. The form of B-12 in supplements is more easily absorbed than naturally occurring B-12.

Pantothenic Acid:

This B vitamin is essential for producing and metabolizing fats. It also helps in the formation of hormones and cholesterol. Pantothenic acid is widely distributed in plant and animal foods. Deficiency is extremely rare.

Biotin:

Biotin is involved in energy production from food and in the metabolism of fatty acids. Deficiency has only been observed in people eating raw eggs. Raw egg contains a substance that interferes with biotin.

You will note that there is some flexibility and safety in taking the B vitamins in greater amounts than the RDA. If your preferred multivitamin/ multi-mineral does not reach your preferred dosage, add a B-complex. Often this is much less expensive than searching for an "all-in-one."

3. Additional Vitamins and Trace Minerals

Vitamin A:

Vitamin A is important for normal vision, health of the skin and cells lining the gastrointestinal tract, gene expression, reproduction, development of the fetus, growth, and immune function. Food sources of vitamin A, as retinol, include liver, kidney, butter, cheese, whole milk, fortified low-fat and skim milk. Vitamin A, in the form of carotenoids, is found in fruits and vegetables.

Because massive amounts of vitamin A can cause birth defects, an Upper Tolerable Intake Level is established for adults. Of the vitamins, the biggest worry for toxicity is vitamin A. Vitamin A is highly concentrated in fish liver and polar bear liver. This is why we caution people against taking more than the dose recommended on the label of the vitamin preparation. Vitamin A in high doses can be dangerous because the body stores excessive amounts of this vitamin. This only applies to retinol. The carotenoids, including beta-carotene, are non-toxic and are converted to vitamin A in the body only when the body requires more vitamin A.

Chromium:

A form of chromium, trivalent chromium, helps insulin in regulating glucose and lipid metabolism. Because of this insulin response, chromium is also thought to be useful for weight loss. Recent studies have shown that chromium picolinate improves insulin sensitivity and glucose use in obese rats. Research is ongoing to determine if this also occurs in humans, as it could be important for those with diabetes. Food sources of chromium include whole grains, meats, dairy products, brewer's yeast, and beer.

Copper:

Copper is needed for the synthesis of hemoglobin, the manufacture of collagen, and the maintenance of the myelin sheath that surrounds nerve fibers. It is also necessary for the proper functioning of the heart. Copper is a part of many enzymes involved in making neurotransmitters. Copper is essential for making superoxide dismutase and glutathione peroxidase. Both enzymes quench free radicals, especially those that damage mitochondria, DNA, fats, and LDL (the bad cholesterol). Food sources of copper are whole grains, liver, kidney, oysters, and nuts. Copper deficiency is rare.

Iodine:

Iodine is an essential component of the thyroid hormones. Deficiencies of iodine lead to goiter (enlarged thyroid) and inadequate thyroid hormone. Thyroid hormone regulates the body's metabolism. Seafood, saltwater fish, and kelp contain iodine. Iodized salt is also available.

Iron:

About 70% of the iron we absorb from the gut is found in hemoglobin, a protein that releases oxygen to body cells for energy production and gives color to red blood cells. Some iron is also found in muscle cells, other proteins, and enzymes. Iron deficiency results in anemia, developmental delays, cognitive impairment, poor pregnancy outcomes, and impaired physical performance.

There are many food sources of iron. The iron contained in meat, fish, and poultry is better absorbed than the iron found in plant sources. Tea and coffee inhibit iron absorption, while vitamin C enhances it.

Manganese:

Manganese is involved in protein and energy metabolism and is essential for normal bone structure. It is also needed for the functioning of the nervous system. Like copper, manganese is involved in producing superoxide dismutase and glutathione peroxidase, which are antioxidants. Manganese is found in legumes and whole grains.

Molybdenum:

Molybdenum has been found to be a component of several of the body's enzymes. Molybdenum occurs in meats, grains, and legumes.

Zinc:

Zinc is an essential component of nearly 100 enzymes, and is the second most abundant trace mineral in the body next to iron. It is required for normal growth and development in children, and is involved in carbohydrate use, making proteins, and replication of DNA. Zinc joins copper and manganese in producing superoxide dismutase and glutathione peroxidase. Zinc is found in meats, poultry, oysters, eggs, and legumes.

Although zinc deficiency is rare, it can occur. Those at risk include male long-distance runners (zinc is lost in the sweat), alcoholics, and vegetarians.

4. The Antioxidant Vitamins and Minerals

Vitamin C:

Vitamin C is a water-soluble antioxidant. In addition, it is a cofactor for enzymes involved in the synthesis of collagen, carnitine, and neurotransmitters. Vitamin C also plays a role in wound healing and resistance to infections. It provides substantial antioxidant protection in the eye, in white blood cells, and in semen. It also protects LDL (the bad cholesterol) from being oxidized and contributing to heart disease. Vitamin C has the ability to recycle other antioxidants such as glutathione and vitamin E. Vitamin C has a protective effect against cancers of the oral cavity, larynx, esophagus, lung, stomach, colon, rectum, and cervix. In addition, vitamin C is involved in iron absorption, transport, and storage.

Vitamin C deficiency is rare in developed countries, but can occur in individuals consuming few fruits and vegetables or in alcoholics. Food sources of vitamin C include vegetables such as broccoli, peppers, potatoes, Brussels sprouts, and fruits such as oranges, cranberries, grapefruit, and plums. Exposure of foods to heat and light reduces the vitamin C content. Also, vitamin C can easily be leached out into the cooking water. Prevent vitamin C losses by covering containers of cut fruits and vegetables and of juices.

The best form of vitamin C supplement is esterified C. Esterified C combines minerals such as calcium, potassium, or zinc with the ascorbic acid. This makes the supplement non-acidic and more readily absorbed by the body.

Vitamin E:

Vitamin E is a fat-soluble antioxidant. It protects fats against oxidation. Vitamin E is found in vegetable and seed oils, nuts and seeds, and green and leafy green vegetables. Excellent sources are wheat germ oil, sunflower and safflower oil, peanuts, almonds, and soybean, corn, and canola oils.

Vitamin E deficiency is rare. Interestingly, the RDA is based only on alpha-tocopherol—the other forms of tocopherol that occur naturally in food are not considered to contribute to vitamin E activity. However, the mode of action and effectiveness of the various forms of vitamin E are not well understood at this time. Further research may well reveal that the other forms of tocopherol also have important functions in the body.

Much research has been done on vitamin E (alpha-tocopherol) to determine its role in disease prevention, and a great deal of controversy exists. The bulk of the evidence does not indicate high levels of vitamin E as being beneficial for heart disease. Vitamin E has been shown to be protective against several cancers, including prostate and colon cancer. It is reasonable to suggest that if a vitamin E supplement is taken, it should be in the range of 300-400 IU/day. We recommend a combination of d-alpha, d-gamma, and tocotrienol.

Selenium:

Selenium is a required component of the enzyme glutathione peroxidase, which provides protection from free radicals. Selenium can regenerate vitamin C. In addition, it is involved the regulation of the thyroid hormone. Selenium protects against toxic doses of the heavy metals cadmium, mercury, and silver. Selenium deficiency has been linked to cancer and heart disease.

Food sources of selenium include Brazil nuts, dairy products, onions, grains, nuts, chicken, meats, and seafood. The selenium content of foods is dependent on the selenium in the soil where the food is grown. People who live on the west coast of North America, particularly British Columbia, Washington, and Oregon, need to be aware that the soil in these areas is selenium depleted. Because of this, it may be prudent to include selenium as a supplement.

Recent studies have demonstrated that supplemental selenium at 200 mcg/day reduces anxiety and depression, and helps to increase energy. It is thought that selenium does this by enhancing dopamine (feel-good) levels in the brain.

Alpha-lipoic Acid, Coenzyme Q-10, and Glutathione:

These antioxidant nutrients are discussed in Chapter 3. Generally speaking, only limited amounts of these are obtained through food. Furthermore, our need for these increase with age, chronic illness, and use of medications. Thus, supplements are well advised.

How Much Do You Need?

Listed in the following chart are the "official" RDA or DRI (daily recommended intake) levels of several important vitamins, minerals, and antioxidants. Also listed are the supplementation levels we recommend. These amounts are *total* daily amounts. In some cases we also list a "treatment" level, which will apply to some individuals with chronic illness or auto-immune disease.

BONE-RELATED NUTRIENTS

	RDA Amount/day	Recommended Daily Supplement	Upper Level of Tolerable Intake
Calcium	1,000 mg/day adults aged 19-50	500 mg/day adults aged 19-50	2,500 mg/day
	1,200 mg/day adults over 50	1,000 mg/day adults over 50	
		1,500 mg/day if risk of osteoporosis	
Phosphorus	700 mg/day	–	4,000 mg/day adults
Magnesium	320 mg/day women	500 mg/day	toxicity level is 800-1,000 mg/day
	420 mg/day men		

	RDA Amount/day	Recommended Daily Supplement	Upper Level of Tolerable Intake
Vitamin D	200 IU/day adults aged 19-50	1,000 IU/day for all adults	2,000 IU/day*
	400 IU/day adults aged 51-70	2,000 IU/day if risk of osteoporosis	
	600 IU/day adults aged 71+	4,000 IU/day if auto-immune disorder or risk of cancer	

Dr. Vieth's research suggests 4,000 IU/day is safe. He states that toxicity for vitamin D is 40,000 IU/day.

Fluoride	3 mg/day women		10 mg/day
	4 mg/day men		
Vitamin K	90 mcg/day women	40 mcg/day	not known
	120 mcg/day men		
Boron	not known	1 mg/day	20 mg/day

THE B VITAMINS

Thiamin (Vit B-1)	1.1 mg/day women	50-100 mg/day if smoker, drinker, work shifts, stressful lifestyle, or chronic illness	not known
	1.2 mg/day men		

	RDA Amount/day	Recommended Daily Supplement	Upper Level of Tolerable Intake
Riboflavin (Vit B-2)	1.1 mg/day women 1.3 mg/day men	same as thiamin	not known
Niacin (Vit B-3)	14 mg/day women 16 mg/day men	same as thiamin	35 mg/day
Pyridoxine (Vit B-6)	1.3 mg/day adults aged 19-50 1.5 mg/day women aged 51+ 1.7 mg/day men aged 51+	50-100 mg/day	100 mg/day
Folate (Folic Acid)	400 mcg/day adults	400 mcg/day	1,000 mcg/day
Vitamin B-12	2.4 mcg/day adults	2.4-6 mcg/day	not known
Pantothenic Acid	5 mg/day adults	5 mg/day	not known
Biotin	30 mcg/day adults	30 mcg/day	not known

ADDITIONAL VITAMINS AND TRACE MINERALS

	RDA Amount/day	Recommended Daily Supplement	Upper Level of Tolerable Intake
Vitamin A	700 mcg/day (2,333 IU retinol) women 900 mcg/day (3,000 IU retinol) men	not recommended but if taken, supplement to level of RDA or less	3,000 mcg/day (10,000 IU/day) Toxicity is a problem.
Carotenoids	none established 10,000-20,000 IU per day of alpha- and beta-carotene, lutein, and lycopene	recommend 5,000-15,000 IU beta-carotene	not known
Chromium	25 mcg/day women 20 mcg/day women aged 51+ 35 mcg/day men aged 19-50 30 mcg/day men aged 51+	200 mcg/day	not known
Copper	900 mcg/day adults	1/10th the level of zinc supplement Example: if 15 mg of zinc, then 1.5 mg of copper	10,000 mcg/day
Iodine	150 mcg/day adults	100-150 mcg/day	1,100 mcg/day

	RDA Amount/day	Recommended Daily Supplement	Upper Level of Tolerable Intake
Iron	18 mg/day women aged 19-50	18 mg/day women aged 19-50	45 mg/day
	8 mg/day women aged 51+	not recommended for men and post-menopausal women	
	8 mg/day men		
Manganese	18 mg/day women aged 19-50	RDA levels	11 mg/day
	8 mg/day men & women aged 51+		
Molybdenum	45 mcg/day adults	45 mcg/day	2,000 mcg/day
Zinc	11 mg/day women	15 mg	40 mg/day
	8 mg/day men		

THE ANTIOXIDANT VITAMINS AND MINERALS

	RDA Amount/day	Recommended Daily Supplement	Upper Level of Tolerable Intake
Vitamin C	75 mg/day women	200-500 mg/day	2,000 mg/day
	95 mg/day men		
Vitamin E	15 mg/day (22 IU/day) adults	200-400 IU/day (1,500 IU/day)	1,000 mg/day
Selenium	55 mcg/day adults	200 mcg/day	400 mcg/day

	RDA Amount/day	Recommended Daily Supplement	Upper Level of Tolerable Intake
Alpha-lipoic Acid	not known	100 mg/day	not known
Coenzyme Q-10	not known	50 mg/day adults over 40 100 mg/day if heart disease	not known
Glutathione	not known	20-40 g/day undenatured whey protein isolate	Safety of whey is well established. Caution in persons with advanced liver or kidney disease.

The information provided in this chapter is only a small amount of what is known about some of the essential vitamins and minerals. Much more could be written—we chose to give you only the basic information. Nutritional science is a young science. Indeed, the first vitamins were only discovered in the early 1900s. Research continues into the roles of nutrients in health and disease. Sometimes the information is contradictory and confusing; other times it is more conclusive. A new area of nutritional research is nutrigenomics, the study of the interaction of nutrients with our genetic material. That is, certain nutrients can turn genes on or off and thus have an impact on our health and the development of disease. Ongoing research will reveal even more exciting information on how foods and nutrients interact in our bodies to promote healing, health, and longevity.

Going into More Detail

Both Health Canada and the Food and Nutrition Board of the Institute of Medicine have led the development of nutrient recommendations in North America. Over time, these have become almost sacrosanct. The knowledge base for these nutritional estimates was based on six criteria:

1. The amount of the particular nutrient that healthy people consume.

2. The amount needed to avoid a particular disease (e.g., scurvy was very common and the recommended daily allowance of vitamin C is enough to prevent scurvy).

3. The degree of tissue saturation or the adequacy of body function in relation to that nutrient intake.

4. Nutrient balance studies that measure nutritional status in relation to intake.

5. Studies of volunteers experimentally maintained on diets deficient in a nutrient, followed by their improvement, or signs of deficiency going away, when a certain amount of the nutrient is re-supplied.

6. Extrapolation from animal experiments in which deficiencies have been produced by exclusion of a single nutrient from the diet.

From 1997 to 2002, a joint committee of experts from Canada and the United States collaborated to produce the Dietary Reference Intakes (DRIs). The DRIs consist of four types of nutrient recommendations for healthy individuals: Adequate Intake (AI), Estimated Average Requirement (EAR), Recommended Dietary Allowance (RDA), and Tolerable Upper Intake Level (UL).

When insufficient scientific information is available for a particular vitamin or mineral, Adequate Intake (AI) is determined. The AI is based on the approximate intake of a nutrient by a group, or groups, of healthy people. For example, the AI for adult men for manganese is 2.3 mg/day. For adult women, the AI is 2 mg/day.

The Estimated Average Requirement (EAR) is the average requirement of a nutrient for healthy individuals—the amount of a nutrient that would meet the needs of half of a given healthy population. Thus, EAR should only be used when assessing the nutrient adequacy of populations, not individuals.

The new RDA is the amount of a nutrient that would meet the requirements of 97-98% of healthy individuals. The RDA then becomes the goal for intake for individuals. It is important to remember that nutrient needs change throughout our lifetimes. What is needed by a child might be very different from what is needed by an adult over 70. For example, the RDA for folate for children ages 1-3 is 150 mcg/day, while the RDA for individuals aged 14 and older is 400 mcg/day.

Tolerable Upper Intake Levels (ULs) have been established to reduce the risk of toxic effects from over-consumption of nutrients. The UL is believed to be the highest level of a nutrient intake that is safe for the specified group. Some feel that the range between the RDA and the UL may represent nutrient intakes that may promote health or prevent disease. Some scientists, health practitioners, and nutrition experts disagree with the RDAs and ULs, and recommend even higher levels of nutrients for disease prevention and treatment of diseases. These higher levels would be considered a "therapeutic" level and would require ongoing supervision and counsel by the practitioner.

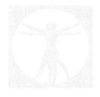

CHAPTER THREE

Antioxidants: Powerful Protection

Most of us credit Dr. Linus Pauling for his early approach to antioxidants, especially for touting the value of vitamin C. Although Dr. Pauling was awarded two Nobel Prizes, he was decried by most physicians and scientists for promoting what they felt was nutritional quackery. Dr. Pauling was a pioneer in nutritional medicine and much of what he promoted has proven to be valid. He believed that nutrition could prevent, help, or cure many diseases. He was one of the first scientists to determine that free radicals, produced by oxidative stress, could damage all of our body tissues. Let us explore the notion of oxidative stress and the source of these free radicals.

Cells: Our Body's Basic Building Blocks

We each have some 70 trillion cells making up all our tissues and organs (e.g., heart, brain, skin, blood, bones, etc). Our circulating blood delivers the nutrients these cells require and carries away the by-products. Each cell must create its own energy from the food we eat and the oxygen we breathe. This blending or mixing of food and oxygen is called oxidation. A wood-burning fire is a superb analogy to the burning of food (fuel) in our bodies. The wood logs represent our food. In order to burn, the fire needs oxygen from the air. The fire releases smoke and carbon dioxide into the air. The heat and light from the fire represent the energy released from the wood.

Just as the fire produces by-products from burning wood for energy, our bodies produce by-products from burning food for energy. When our cells use food for fuel, heat is produced, little packets of energy known as ATP (Adenosine TriPhosphate) are made, and carbon dioxide is given off by our lungs. This compares to the heat and light energy and the carbon dioxide from the wood fire.

What do the by-products of smoke and ashes from the fire represent in our bodies? These are the *free radicals* released from the mitochondria, the cell's power center. Whenever our bodies use oxygen in a process called oxidation, unstable molecules—free radicals—are formed. Indeed, tens of thousands of free radicals are produced naturally in the body every day. A free radical can start a chain reaction in its frenzy to become stable, making other molecules unstable. Thus, anything in the way of free radicals—such as proteins, fats, and DNA—can be damaged. Excess free radicals must be stopped. Nature's solution to this problem is antioxidants, which trap free radicals and stop the domino effects of their damage to cells.

What Contributes to Free Radical Excess?

- *Polluted air and water*
- *Herbicides and pesticides in food*
- *Trans fats in foods*
- *Any drugs—more drugs result in more toxins*
- *Exercise, especially intensive training*
- *Insufficient fruits and vegetables*
- *Smoking*

Exercise and the Use of Energy

We know that when we exercise we breathe deeper and quicker and that our heart beats faster to supply extra oxygen to our muscle cells. Extra food (calories) is also required. The carbon dioxide is readily breathed out. This burst of oxidation (energy production) produces the extra energy our muscle cells require. As a result of this increased production of energy, a large number of free radicals are released into our muscle cells. These excess free radicals are experienced as physical discomfort in the form of muscle stiffness and soreness over the next 12-36 hours. Thus, exercise is a simple example of "oxidative stress." Irritated muscle cells cry out for their excess free radicals to be "quenched." This is why antioxidants are so important. They are able to deal with the reactive, damaging free radicals and render them harmless.

If we "super train," as an Olympic athlete would need to, then this excess of free radicals must be dealt with by optimal nutrition and nutrition supplements. If not, the heightened free radicals exhaust our cells' antioxidants, including glutathione, found in our white blood cells. The result is a depressed immune system. Hence we are more vulnerable to infections such as colds or flu viruses at the time of peak training for competition. Most of us can recall a favorite Olympic athlete who was not performing optimally as a consequence.

Another example of oxidative stress is a partly eaten apple. The exposed fleshy part turns brown over a few hours, due to oxidation. This oxidative stress is precipitated or caused by oxygen contacting the exposed apple. The browning is due to free radical excess. To avoid the browning, we can dip the exposed apple in lemon juice. The vitamin C in this citrus fruit quenches the free radicals and solves the oxidative stress by supplying an antioxidant.

The Cell and Oxidative Stress

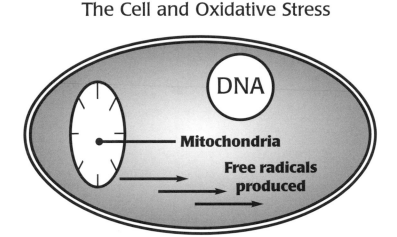

The Cell and Oxidative Stress: The outside double lining represents our double-layered lipid (fat) cell membrane. DNA is inside the nucleus of the cell. The small egg-shaped oval represents the mitochondria, or power center, which produces energy within the cell. Each cell has many mitochondria to fuel body activity.

What is it in the cell that is similar to the apple edges turning brown? Following is an outline as well as three different examples of how excess free radicals act in the cells (i.e., oxidative stress). First, excess free radicals injure the DNA (deoxyribonucleic acid), which is the blueprint for new cells, DNA, and proteins. Injured DNA markedly increases our risk of cancer. Our body produces thousands of new cancer cells daily. Excess free radicals compound or increase this cancer-cell production. Certainly, those of us with chronic pain or MS do not need another strike against our health to slow us down on our journey to recovery!

Second, excess free radicals injure our cell membranes, which are made of a double layer of fat (lipid). The cell membrane protects each individual cell and controls what passes into the cell and what the cell releases. If excess free radicals damage the cell membrane, the cell loses its protective membrane control and good and bad components can travel easily in and out of the cell. Inevitably, the cell is injured and dies early. This is a key step in premature aging.

We are actually genetically programmed to live healthy and well to 120-140 years. Changes in hygiene, sanitation, and food have improved our chances of this. Unfortunately, the downhill slide of our SAD (Standard American Diet) has increased our chronic and fatal diseases and thereby shortened our life as well. Most of us are dying prematurely in our 60s, 70s, or 80s due to degenerative diseases such as heart disease, cancer, stroke, and diabetes. Research confirms that degenerative diseases are induced by oxidative stress. Therefore, we hope to encourage the trend of "whole food junkies." All of us need to consume more "whole foods" such as fruits, vegetables, seeds, nuts, and legumes and fewer processed foods full of salt, sugar, and trans fat and devoid of vitamins and minerals and much reduced in phytonutrients (plant chemicals).

The third part of the cell injured due to free radical excess is the mitochondria or "power center." Oxidative stress from excess free radicals reduces this power center's ability to produce energy. This is a key factor in a lack of energy in general, and in illnesses such as chronic fatigue syndrome and fibromyalgia (in Europe called fibromyositis), and probably accounts for the fatigue of MS, rheumatoid arthritis, systemic lupus erythematosus, and advanced cancers.

More about Stress and Stress Protection

After the above discussion on free radicals and oxidative stress, you can perhaps see how Dr. Linus Pauling was well ahead of his time. Similarly, endocrinologist Hans Selye's concepts of emotional, mental, and physical stress have been verified. Excessive mental and emotional stress greatly increases free radical production. Pollutants in our air, food, and water, cigarette smoke, sunlight, and fatty meals (which also contain trans fats) all increase our production of free radicals. Even medications, chemotherapy, and radiation treatments, given in an effort to fight disease, produce free radicals as the body strives to deal with their aftereffects. Exercise, especially when done excessively, exponentially increases the production of free radicals.

Our favorite example when discussing oxidative stress is airplane travel in excess of four hours. The triggers of extra free radicals are: reduced oxygen, shared air and viruses, and ever-increasing radiation exposure the higher we fly. My recommendation: when you must take an airplane, boost your vitamin C intake with at least a 500 mg supplement. Also, increase your fruits and vegetables as much as possible for the vitamin C and the phytonutrients, which are subtle but powerful antioxidants.

In order to protect our health, now more than ever, we need to reduce the things that produce free radicals and optimize our antioxidant protection. We can never be free of the damaging free radicals, but we can protect ourselves with a blend of antioxidants and then repair oxidative damage with the necessary nutritional building blocks.

For example, did you know that while a whole apple has about 8 mg of vitamin C, it also contains dozens of phytonutrients? These phytonutrients have an antioxidant ability equal to 600 mg of vitamin C. The "apple a day keeps the doctor away" saying of our childhood was correct after all! By eating more fruits and vegetables, you will recover health, help anti-aging, and potentially reach optimal health.

In order to protect our health, now more than ever, we need to reduce the things that produce free radicals and optimize our antioxidant protection. We can never be free of the damaging free radicals, but we can protect ourselves with a blend of antioxidants and then repair oxidative damage with the necessary nutritional building blocks.

Antioxidants are either made in the body or obtained from food or nutritional supplements. Antioxidants made by the body include glutathione, alpha-lipoic acid, and Coenzyme Q-10 (CoQ-10). Of all the antioxidants in the body, glutathione is the "master" antioxidant and is discussed more fully in the next chapter. However, most of our antioxidants are obtained from food—another good reason to eat a healthy diet! Vitamin C, vitamin E, plus carotenoids and flavonoids from plants are found naturally in foods. We can also obtain antioxidants from nutritional supplements.

Alpha-lipoic acid is both fat soluble and water soluble. This enables lipoic acid to fight free radicals anywhere in the body. Alpha-lipoic acid can also work with vitamins C and E and with glutathione to rejuvenate them. This antioxidant has many roles in the body—it prevents LDL (bad cholesterol) oxidation and reduces growth of cancer cells, as well as aids the immune system. In addition, alpha-lipoic acid bonds with toxic metals and therefore helps detoxify the body. For maximum free radical protection, a supplement containing alpha-lipoic acid is recommended. Dr. Lester Packer, a world authority on antioxidants, recommends a level of 100 mg/day of alpha-lipoic acid supplement.

Coenzyme Q-10 (CoQ-10), which can be made in the body, helps the body produce energy. This is especially important in the high-energy areas of the body—the heart, brain, kidneys, and liver. As an antioxidant, CoQ-10 works to prevent free radical damage in fatty tissues including the brain and the other high-energy areas of the body. Unfortunately, our CoQ-10 production declines with age.

The Japanese have long used CoQ-10 for the treatment of heart disease. It is now known that drugs for lowering cholesterol deplete the body of CoQ-10. Hence people on these drugs, or those with heart disease, would benefit from CoQ-10 supplementation. Also, recent studies reveal that people on anti-depressants should also supplement their CoQ-10, for similar reasons.

CoQ-10 is found in food such as organ meats and salmon. Dr. Packer states that it is nearly impossible to get enough CoQ-10 from diet alone. He recommends a CoQ-10 supplement of 50 mg/day for adults over 40 years of age. For people with heart disease, he recommends an additional 50 mg/day.

Vitamin C, our best-known and one of the first-discovered antioxidants, is water soluble. Thus it acts in the blood and within the fluid of the cells. The vitamin C in limes, when fed to sailors, prevented "scurvy." Sailors, after months at sea, and lacking fresh fruits or vegetables, became deficient in vitamin C. In fact, the DRI (Dietary Reference Intake) for vitamin C (90 mg/day for adult males and 75 mg/day for adult females) is enough to stop scurvy, with a small safety margin. This does not, however, tell us how much is needed for optimal health, for prevention of chronic disease, or to counteract a sudden burst in extra free radicals. Linus Pauling and many other health and nutrition practitioners (including us) recommend an intake of vitamin C far more than the DRI, ranging from 500 mg/day to 1-2 g/day.

Vitamin C plays an important role in protecting the cell's mitochondria. It can neutralize free radicals before they injure the mitochondria. Vitamin C also boosts the activity of other antioxidants, especially vitamin E. When vitamin E quenches a free radical, it becomes a free radical itself. Vitamin C can then react with the vitamin E to restore it. Scientists have recently discovered that vitamin E can regenerate vitamin C too. Maintaining our levels of vitamins C and E allows continuous regeneration. This is truly a synergistic partnership.

Certainly our second best-known antioxidant is vitamin E. It is a fat-soluble antioxidant and plays an important role in protecting the cell membrane from free radical damage. It is also a component of LDL, the "lousy" or "bad" form of blood cholesterol. Vitamin E has a role in preventing oxidation of LDL and damage to the cells that line blood vessel walls. Both LDL oxidation and blood vessel damage lead to plaque buildup and progression of heart disease. Evidence also exists that vitamin E protects the body against aging, arthritis, cancer, cataracts, diabetes, and infection. The DRI for vitamin E is 15 mg/day (22 IU). Again, many health and nutrition practitioners recommend doses of vitamin E in excess of the DRI. However, too much vitamin E can be a problem. Recent studies report that vitamin E beyond 400 IU can be harmful. Therefore, an upper limit of 400 IU is recommended as a supplement. Further individual discussion on vitamins and minerals is in Chapter 2.

An important discovery is that vitamins C and E, alpha-lipoic acid, CoQ-10, and glutathione are network antioxidants—meaning they work together in the body to enhance our health and protect us from disease. Together these antioxidants work more effectively and enhance the antioxidant protection. Therefore, they are thought to be especially effective in protecting us from disease and aging.

Another group of antioxidants is the flavonoid group. There are more than 4,000 flavonoids found in plants, but the plant foods we commonly eat contain 50 flavonoids. These substances give plants their bright colors and protect the plants from diseases. Plants have been used by humans for thousands of years for their medicinal properties. Research has confirmed that flavonoids are important to our health. Besides being antioxidants, the flavonoids improve memory and concentration, boost the effectiveness of vitamin C, reduce inflammation, improve immune function, and protect us from heart disease.

For these reasons, ginkgo biloba, pycnogenol from pine bark, apples, berries, citrus fruits, cruciferous vegetables (broccoli, cauliflower, kale, cabbage and Brussels sprouts), garlic, onions, green leafy vegetables, grapes, wine, soy, tea, walnuts, turmeric, milk thistle, and grapeseed extract are rich sources of flavonoids. We encourage everyone to include these in his or her diet as often as possible.

Carotenoids are another class of antioxidants obtained from plants. Carotenoids are found in many fruits and vegetables. They are fat soluble and are absorbed best in the body in the presence of dietary fat. Over 600 carotenoids exist, but only a few are nutritionally significant. Carotenoids are partly responsible for many of the well-documented health benefits of diets rich in fruits and vegetables.

Carotenoids have many health benefits. Because they protect DNA from free radical damage, they play a role in cancer prevention. For example, diets high in lycopene and high blood levels of lycopene are associated with decreased risk of prostate cancer. Beta-carotene and lycopene protect the skin from ultraviolet (UV) radiation damage. Lutein works to prevent cataracts and macular degeneration. Lutein and lycopene protect against cardiovascular diseases. Sources of lycopene include tomatoes, pink grapefruit, and watermelon. Leafy green vegetables such as spinach, kale, and chard, egg yolks, and dark fruits contain lutein. At this time, no RDA has been established for carotenoids.

Eating for Protection

No one antioxidant can protect the body from all free radicals. Because such a wide variety of antioxidants exists in our food supply, aim to eat a variety of different plant foods every day. This means you should eat 8-10 servings of fruits and vegetables every day. (The average North American only eats 2-3 servings of fruits and vegetables daily. A serving is a ½-cup portion of fruit, vegetable, or juice.) In fact, in 2005, the U.S. government revised the Dietary Guidelines for Americans to include *more* fruits and vegetables. Americans are now encouraged to eat 2 cups of fruits per day and 2½ cups of vegetables. This amount is based on a 2,000-calorie diet for adults and reflects 4 servings of fruit and 5 servings of vegetables.

Americans are now encouraged to eat 2 cups of fruits per day and 2½ cups of vegetables.

Canadians should take note: Health Canada is currently reviewing Canada's Food Guide, and, no doubt, recommendations will be forthcoming that also encourage more fruits and vegetables.

Eating lots of fruits and vegetables, especially brightly colored ones, will provide your body with many different antioxidants. The overall benefits will be greater than if you only have a few antioxidants. Select antioxidant supplements to complement your intake of antioxidants from food. Science cannot yet tell us what level of antioxidant protection we need individually.

However, there is overwhelming evidence for the role of antioxidants in promoting health, preventing chronic diseases, and treating illness.

In recognition of the health benefits of antioxidants, many products now appear on store shelves. Capsules with dried fruit and vegetable mixtures, plant-based powders, fruit and vegetable bars, juices, and many other plant-based supplements are now available. As with all products, consumers beware. Quality varies, as do components. Many consumers are bewildered by the choices. Make sure to read labels and check out the proportions of the various ingredients. Read promotional materials carefully. Ask the same questions you would ask when choosing vitamin/mineral supplements. You can review these in the chapter on vitamins and minerals.

Nature provides us with an exciting array of plants. Science will continue to reveal the different components in plants and how they contribute to our health. Even if we do not yet understand how these phytonutrients, or plant chemicals, work in our bodies, one thing we know for sure: We know that we should eat plenty of fruits and vegetables, especially the brightly colored ones. They are our passports to vibrant health.

Measuring Our Intake

As humans looking for evidence or proof, we like to measure things and have objective information. This is especially true as it applies to our health. We measure our height, weight, blood pressure, cholesterol, and blood sugar in order to evaluate our health. We might question our iron, B-12, or vitamin D status. People often wonder, too, if they are getting enough vitamins and minerals. Levels of these can be obtained from blood samples.

In summary, our bodies are subjected to free radicals that are produced internally and those that result from exposure to our external environment—our air, water, and food. We can optimize our dietary intake, including supplements, or optimize our stress, air, water, food, and environment. We are now in "control" of our well-being, and we truly "are what we (swallow or) eat."

CHAPTER FOUR

Glutathione: Master Antioxidant/#1 Detoxifier

Glutathione (GSH) is the body's master antioxidant and is found in every body cell. It is a small protein that is produced naturally in the body from three amino acids (glycine, glutamine, and cysteine). GSH is essential to life—without it, we die. The scientific literature has over 50,000 articles discussing GSH and its importance to health. Indeed, this tiny protein is known as the body's essential health "AID" for its **A**ntioxidant protection, **I**mmune system modulation, and ability to **D**etoxify the body.

GSH is a new concept. Most people are not aware of its role in health, and most health professionals have only a vague idea of its importance. Soon, GSH will become common knowledge, much as cholesterol and blood sugar are today. All healthcare practitioners, including physicians, will want to know the glutathione levels of their patients. Why will this happen? GSH levels are an indicator of health and of how long a person will live.

Currently, GSH measurement is done by a blood sample and reflects GSH concentration in the body over several weeks. The red blood cells are frozen to break down the cell membrane, and hence the measurement of GSH reflects the concentration inside the cell, or its cytoplasmic concentration. The test costs approximately $40-$100. Red blood cell GSH represents an average over 120 days and hence a more ideal measurement would be white blood cell GSH.

The importance of GSH was reported in a 2004 *New England Journal of Medicine*. Glutathione peroxidase (an enzyme in the glutathione building pathway) was touted as being the best predictor of a heart attack—surpassing C-reactive protein (CRP). (Elevated levels of CRP are found in people with heart disease.) GSH and glutathione peroxidase are directly related. Neither will be produced in excess in the body, as each has a major protective feedback loop to prevent this. In the future, GSH measurement, as a health indicator, will supersede cholesterol, C-reactive protein, the ESR (Erythrocyte Sedimentation Rate) and probably glutathione peroxidase.

Still, we are relatively unable to raise our body's intracellular GSH with regular food, GSH capsules, or even n-acetyl-cysteine (NAC) by mouth. Considerable GSH is present in many fruits, vegetables, and meats, but it is digested before the body can make use of it. GSH is digested into its three amino acids: glycine, glutamine, and cysteine. Cysteine, alone in the gut after GSH digestion, is a sulfur-containing amino acid and is treated as a free radical. It is almost immediately oxidized to a charged molecule. Very little of this single, charged cysteine amino acid is able to pass through the gut lining into our bloodstream. Hence, an optimal supplement must be able to deliver bioactive cysteine all the way to the cells. Certain whey protein isolates likely maintain the three-dimensional protein structure, permitting an excellent cysteine delivery system. Other key amino acids, such as leucine, may also be synergistic in optimal formation of GSH in the cell. This three-dimensional structure is largely why individual amino acids, or mixtures of amino acids, are less potent or effective than nature's plan— undenatured whey protein isolates.

NAC, if given by mouth, is only slightly more successful in raising general body cells' GSH. Only 6-10% is absorbed through the gut and very little is taken up into the body cells. Almost zero NAC is able to cross the blood-brain barrier. This is indeed unfortunate, as many brain illnesses are worsened due to the lack of GSH inside brain cells.

What would we find if we measured blood GSH in those people with brain illnesses, particularly MS? By the time a person has been diagnosed with either MS or Parkinson's, both neurodegenerative diseases, the body's cellular GSH is only 5% of what it should be. Similarly, limited brain GSH is key in the development of ALS and Alzheimer's. In addition, the severity of injury from stroke, brain injury, or brain trauma is greatly affected by brain cell GSH.

The story of the best way to raise GSH in our body's cells is entertaining, exciting, and all Canadian. It began with the immigration from Italy of surgeon Dr. Gustavo Bounous. Dr. Bounous became a lab-based researcher, first in Indiana, then in Sherbrooke, Quebec, Canada, and finally settled in Montreal, Quebec, Canada, at McGill University. In 1967, Dr. Bounous and his associate received a Gold Medal from the Royal College of Physicians and Surgeons of Canada for groundbreaking research in human nutrition. His discovery led to his being funded by the Medical Research Council of Canada. Dr. Bounous was the researcher who developed the "elemental" diet of simple amino acids, fatty acids, and sugars that was tolerated by patients recovering after a major surgery or in intensive care. Dr. Bounous continued his quest for the optimal protein diet to recover from any major body stress.

One day, a box of pure whey protein arrived on his desk from a Swiss dairy company, with a cheque attached. The dairy company hoped Dr. Bounous could determine a medical or economic use for their whey. Whey was a very common by-product of European cheese production.

Rather fortuitously, at this time Dr. Bounous was doing some collaborative studies with Dr. Patricia Kongshavn, an internationally recognized immunology professor at McGill University. They were investigating the effect of using different amino acid ratios in the diet on immune function. When they fed the whey protein to laboratory mice, they found that the animals developed a much stronger immune response when challenged with an antigen than did mice fed any other dietary protein. The whey protein also gave the mice immunity against salmonellosis. Further studies revealed that this whey protein protected the mice against colon cancer. Even more astounding was the finding by Drs. Bounous and Kongshavn that, when the whey protein was given to their laboratory mice, they lived 30-50% longer than when they consumed other equivalent protein diets.

Drs. Bounous and Kongshavn then began working on the method or mechanism of why this whey protein isolate was so unique. However, about this time, their lab experiments quit working. They were still receiving the whey protein from the same company in Europe, sent by the same courier. For the next 30 months, they were unable to reproduce the previous results.

Then, serendipity intervened. While watching television one evening, Dr. Bounous learned that 30 months previously, a salmonella outbreak had occurred in Europe. Subsequent to this, the European health authorities had raised the minimum pasteurization temperature by 3°C. Dr. Bounous felt that the slight rise in pasteurization temperature might be responsible for the lack of results. He could barely wait to resume his research with a North American whey protein isolate, which might enable him to restart his studies. Indeed, it worked!

About this time, Drs. Bounous and Kongshavn then combined their respective talents and energies to unlock the secrets of this whey protein isolate and how it worked in our bodies. They determined that any fresh or carefully pasteurized source of mammalian whey isolate could have profound benefit. For those intuitive among us, this would fit with our premise that fresh breast milk is the optimal food for human babies.

Drs. Bounous and Kongshavn went on to find that 10 grams (0.3 ounce) of white powder from this whey protein isolate could be obtained from one liter (U.S. quart) of human breast milk. The process used to obtain the whey protein isolate was patented (US Patent #5,451,412). These researchers demonstrated that 4-5 liters or 4-5 quarts of cow's milk was needed to produce 10 grams (0.3 ounces) of the same whey protein isolate. This disparity is due to human breast milk being 60% whey protein and 40% casein (cheese) protein; meanwhile, cow's (sheep's, goat's, etc.) milk is 20% whey and 80% casein. The milk is pasteurized at the lowest possible temperature and then micro-filtered through a ceramic unit to further eliminate any bacteria.

All milk is obtained from strictly vegetarian cows, including testing to eliminate milk containing antibiotics or hormones to enhance milk production. The whey is the most desired product in this instance. Casein is removed and sold as a by-product to a cheese company. Similarly, all the fat (fatty acids) are removed and almost all the lactose (sugar). This permits most of us to take this specialized whey protein isolate, a white powder, without lactase enzymes. However, the extremely lactose sensitive should take lactase alone or with a plant digestive enzyme containing lactase.

What is so special about this patented whey protein? Dr. Bounous' theory is that the most unique component is "bonded cysteine," which is maintained within it. This bonded cysteine consists of two cysteine amino acids (which contain sulfur) held together by a "gentle" but all-important disulfide bond. What is a disulfide bond? A good illustration is something we frequently experience in our own hair. Each hair is a strand of protein. Freshly washed hair tends to flatten after two or three days. This "flatness" results from the many, many disulfide bonds or bridges that have formed between strands of hair over that time. How do we "break" most of these bridges? We apply water and shampoo, rinse with water, and towel dry. Now our hair is fluffy again. With this example can see how easy it is to "break" this gentle disulfide bond.

This "bonded cysteine," uniquely present in all fresh mammalian milk, has several special properties. First, it is protected from digestion in the gut by our own digestive enzymes, pepsin and trypsin. Second, this bonded cysteine is a neutral or uncharged molecule and readily passes through the gut lining into our bloodstream. The heart circulates this blood, rich in bonded cysteine, to all body tissues, including the brain. Yes, this bonded cysteine also crosses the blood-brain barrier. Once this uncharged particle is in the fluid surrounding our cells, it readily enters all of our cells. The bonded cysteine supplies two cysteine molecules, both of which are able to combine with glycine and glutamine to form GSH.

Drs. Bounous and Kongshavn and other researchers have now learned that the rate-limiting raw material for the production of GSH inside the cell is cysteine. Each cell's own enzymes readily cleave the bonded cysteine's disulfide bond and this problem is now solved. In addition, the cell will never make more GSH than it needs due to the protective and carefully regulated feedback loop of GSH production. We now know GSH is also an important way for the body to store this critical cysteine amino acid. In fact, in the journal *FASEB* in 2001, Dr. Wulf Dröge described how the cysteine molecule is the critical controller of protein energy malnutrition—and of our healing process!

GSH (glutathione) inside the body has three key functions as previously mentioned. The acronym AID describes this quite well: "A" is for antioxidant, "I" is for immune system modulation or fine-tuning, and "D" is for detoxification.

This is also a very significant piece of the puzzle in healing issues for the person with MS and/or other neurodegenerative illnesses. Certainly, boosting one's intake of bonded cysteine with four packets (10 g each) daily of this "legal white powder" will heal almost any bed sore or "pressure ulcer" within 30-90 days, when added to regular wound care techniques. You see, the skin is the "mirror" of the body's well-being. Therefore, if the skin wound can heal, so will other tissues. This includes muscle cells and even brain cells. Similarly, the body always heals with inflammation (redness, swelling, heat, and pain or loss of function), and optimal GSH also fine-tunes or minimizes inflammation. The cause or trigger of this inflammation includes trauma, surgery, infection, auto-immune illness, and even premature aging. Subsequently, swelling (heat, redness, and pain too) is less, healing is faster, and scar formation is also minimized. This means less acute symptoms of MS, secondary to the swelling of inflammation, with our most obvious being a change in vision. In addition, it reduces the need for a "pulse" of intravenous corticosteroids to control the inflammation of an MS attack.

GSH (glutathione) inside the body has three key functions as previously mentioned. The acronym *AID* describes this quite well: "A" is for antioxidant, "I" is for immune system modulation or fine-tuning, and "D" is for detoxification. GSH is our number one, or master, antioxidant and must be made inside the cell. If adequate GSH can be made inside the cell, it can minimize excess free radical injury to 1) the DNA, and hence reduces cancer; 2) the cell membrane, prolonging cell life and therefore anti-aging; and 3) the mitochondria or power center of the cell, which enhances energy production within the cell. It is this last feature that has enabled Dr. Bill to recover most of his energy and helped give him much of his life back. Today's "energy illnesses" such as chronic fatigue syndrome, fibromyalgia, and probably also the fatigue of MS, rheumatoid arthritis, lupus, and most debilitating illnesses can be improved by raising the GSH inside the cells.

It is now understood that adequate or optimal GSH inside the cells can "recycle" or rejuvenate both vitamins C and E. Hence, Dr. Bill currently supplements with only 300 units of vitamin E and 500 mg of vitamin C daily. Previously, he had to "guess" how much he needed for optimal quenching of free radicals. This also optimizes the body's use of other antioxidants such as Coenzyme Q-10, alpha-lipoic acid, and others.

The Cell and Oxidative Stress

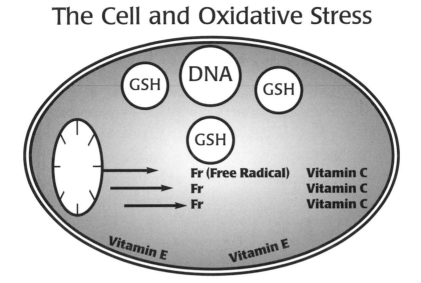

Although not drawn to scale, the above diagram depicts the GSH molecules, which are primarily inside the cell. Without enough GSH in the cell, each vitamin C or E molecule must combine with a free radical and take it all the way out of the body. Whenever there is adequate GSH in the cell, then both vitamin C and E molecules can combine with a free radical, drop the free radical off at the GSH, go and get another, and so on. Now, the cells are able to recycle their vitamin C and E, so less guesswork is needed as to how much to supplement these vitamins. Also, a GSH molecule can combine with a heavy metal (e.g., mercury or lead) and remove that toxin from the body. GSH does similar clearing of drugs once they have acted on the cell receptors and done their job.

Optimal function of the immune system, or white blood cells, is also dependent on the GSH inside these cells. We now realize that the GSH can fall to one-half of optimal in just four to five hours. So, if we optimize this GSH inside our white blood cells, several key changes occur. Our white blood cells act in two major groups: B-cells and T-cells.

B-cells, or humoral white blood cells, are responsible for making our antibody proteins. These attack and combine with foreign proteins or body proteins the body *thinks* are foreign. This is the basis of most of our allergic response (such as hay fever and even asthma) and our auto-immune diseases such as MS, rheumatoid arthritis, lupus, inflammatory bowel diseases, type-1 juvenile onset diabetes, and so on.

T-cells are primarily responsible for cell-mediated immunity within our body. This is the white blood cell function of attacking bacteria, viruses, fungi, cancer cells, and even the antigen-antibody complexes created by the humoral or B-cells. It is now understood that this shift toward cell-mediated immunity from humoral or antigen-antibody immunity reduces not only our hypersensitivity or hyperactive allergic response but also the severity of our auto-immune diseases.

For those of us with a chronic illness such as MS, this also permits fewer bacterial infections such as bladder infections and sinusitis. Similarly, the raised GSH in the brain cells (neurons, astrocytes) and in cells surrounding a neuron being attacked by our own white blood cells will minimize the free radicals produced, thereby injuring a small area rather than a large one. We'll try to explain how this enhanced GSH in our white blood cells modulates their function, rather than simply boosting it.

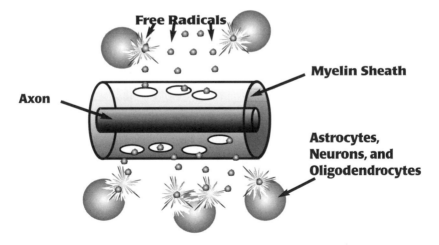

The dark central core represents the nerve's axon. The shaded area around it represents the myelin sheath. The white ovals, seven of them, represent our own white blood cells attacking the myelin. The tiny, shaded circles represent free radicals given off. The large circles represent the surrounding astrocytes, neurons, and oligodendrocytes, which become injured upon contact with the free radicals.

The idea of "boosting" the immune system, per se, will frighten many of us lay people and even some physicians. Heretofore, the understanding of auto-immune illness was as an "overactive" immune system. For example, once Dr. Bill was diagnosed with MS, his physician suggested he stay away from echinacea. Her anxiety was based on the premise that because echinacea boosted his immune system, it could worsen the MS. Happily, this is not a problem, as the "simple" boost is more correctly understood as a modulation, fine-tuning, or even optimization of our white blood cell function. Therefore, it helps relieve rather than aggravate the auto-immune illness. We feel raising Dr. Bill's GSH is one of the biggest pieces (30%) of his MS recovery puzzle. It could have a similar benefit in your pain, MS, or other auto-immune disease journey.

Before finishing our discussion on this GSH-enhancing, key building block whey protein isolate, we want to comment on its safety. It is a food. The U.S. government has granted it GRAS status (i.e., generally regarded as safe). People who are sensitive to, or allergic to, this "humanized" milk protein are rare—only one person in 100,000 has a true whey protein allergy. Also, for the last five years it has been listed as a dietary supplement for cancer and AIDS in the Physician's Desk Reference (PDR) and the Pharmacist's Red Book—key standard texts in the United States. (See *Appendix A & B.*)

In recent months, a new whey protein isolate has been developed to enhance brain function and recovery. (See *Appendix A & B.*) This formula is designed for physicians helping clients taper off anti-anxiety and anti-depressant medications. This mixture includes several B vitamins, selenium, zinc, and vitamin D—all key for optimal brain health. We were both involved in developing this particular formulation.

What did we do when we first learned about building up GSH with these 10-g (0.3–oz.) packets of the whey protein isolate? We started carefully, and cheaply, of course! This meant one packet per day, mixed in fruit juice, water, milk, yogurt, or applesauce. In addition, we learned *not to heat it* (especially not above 140°F or 55°C) and *not to mix it* in a blender, as this might break the very important bridges of "bonded cysteine." Our new friend Mike, who had introduced the idea to Dr. Bill, also mixed Dr. Bill's first packet at our kitchen table! Mike stirred the powder in a small amount of orange juice with a fork. He then added a little more orange juice.

We then proceeded to try to mix our own, daily for two days. Luckily, Mike phoned back two days later asking how it was going. "It's not!" we replied. Mixing the powder was a real hassle, so we had given up. Plan B, and then Plan C, was presented. Plan B, which was low tech, consisted of a shaker cup, not unlike one used to start making a gravy paste. Plan C, which was "hi-tech," used a tiny, handheld mixer, held below the liquid level of the powder (or else it goes everywhere, quickly!). Both methods work quite adequately, but a spoon helps consume the bubbled froth or lumps. We have also since discovered that a bit of fat from oil or cream can help minimize lumps.

Now that a safe, effective means exists for raising GSH in the body, we recommend that anyone with a chronic illness try this specialized whey protein isolate. It may take two packages, or more, over a 6-month period to experience any benefit. But the health benefits far outweigh the difficulty in mixing and the expense of buying this "white powder." Taking an amount of this whey protein isolate every day has been key to the recovery of Dr. Bill's energy, lost because of his MS. While we must insist that this is not a magic bullet (there are no magic bullets in medicine or nutrition), we do believe that this discovery of the building blocks of glutathione is the most significant step forward in our healthcare since penicillin was discovered.

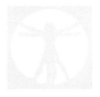

CHAPTER FIVE

Vitamin D: More Than Sunshine

One of the most underrated and least-understood nutrients is vitamin D, the "sunshine vitamin." For years, vitamin D has only been associated with strong bones and teeth. However, over the past 10 years, some fascinating information regarding the many roles of vitamin D has surfaced. Most health professionals, including dieticians and physicians, either have not heard this information or, if they have, they have greeted it with a great deal of skepticism. We strongly believe that vitamin D is a key piece in recovery and optimal health, and we give credit to those brave and wise scientists who have started the vitamin D ball rolling. It is a message that everyone needs to pay attention to. But first, here is some background information.

A comprehensive review by Oliver Gillie called "Sunlight Robbery" describes the link between vitamin D and evolution, and the strong association between inadequate vitamin D and chronic illness. As evidence, he cites over 200 scientific documents. Humans have always needed vitamin D, and this need was demonstrated as changing skin color as our ancestors moved away from the equator and to the north and to the south. At the equator, the dark-skinned people had ample sunshine year-round to make vitamin D in their skin. As they moved from the equator, they received adequate sunlight on bare skin for only part of the year. Consequently, people developed lighter skin to allow for greater vitamin D production during the time that sunshine was effective. Keep in mind that given the same sunlight exposure, pale skin makes vitamin D six times faster than dark skin does. Vitamin D is linked to fertility, thus it was the paler-skinned children who were able to grow and be healthy.

We now know that in midsummer at the 49th parallel (along the U.S.-Canada border) a "white-skinned" person with short sleeves and no hat makes 10,000 units of vitamin D in 20 minutes. Similarly, a dark-brown- or black-skinned person requires 40-60 minutes to make the same amount of vitamin D. You may already be ahead of us in realizing that Northern Europeans (the "hotbed" of MS) such as Scandinavians in Norway, Sweden, Denmark, and Finland, and Celts in Ireland and Scotland, are often very fair-skinned. This change would have occurred relatively quickly, over thousands of years, due to the impact of vitamin D concentration on fertility. This was truly "the survival of the fittest."

Vitamin D is fat soluble. Hence, the fat in the body can maintain it for up to two months, but very little beyond this. This explains why Embry, Snowdon, and Vieth in the annals of *Neurology*, August 2000, noted that MS symptoms and MS lesions or changes on MRI in people in Germany with MS have seasonal fluctuations.

WHY IS INADEQUATE VITAMIN D STILL A MAJOR ISSUE?

1. *Many people live far from the equator.*

2. *In northern areas, there is a lack of UV-B radiation for several months of the year.*

3. *Use of sunscreen blocks the sun's rays from making vitamin D in the skin.*

4. *People limit their exposure to the sun because of the fear of skin cancer.*

5. *Food sources of vitamin D are limited. Therefore, dietary intake is inadequate*

They noted that within two months of the end of their summer (mid or late September) the MS patients were having relapses. Van de Mei and colleagues (2001) also demonstrated that MS prevalence in various regions in Australia was dependent on the ultraviolet radiation. They found a close association between theoretical prevalence predicted from ultraviolet radiation levels (sunshine) and actual MS prevalence.

Work by Vieth in Canada has further enhanced our knowledge of vitamin D and its safety. In the *American Journal of Clinical Nutrition* (1999), he determined that Canadians in their 50s and 60s could readily and safely take 4,000 IU of vitamin D-3 (cholecalciterol) daily for six months. Happily, none of their vitamin D-3 measurements exceeded mid-range. Similarly, Dr. Bill has taken 4,000 IU of vitamin D-3 daily for six years and his vitamin D-3 measures 99—normal range being 30-150 nmol/l. This amount of vitamin D daily sounds less ominous if translated to milligrams, where it is 0.1 mg daily. People with gut absorption concerns, especially fat, may need to take more. We have a colleague who, after taking 4,000 IU/day for five years, found her vitamin D-3 measured only 30.

Current estimates for optimal blood levels of vitamin D-3 to minimize MS symptoms are 90-110 nmol/l. In four studies, 10,000 IU/day (250 mcg) orally of vitamin D-3 is equivalent to full-skin-body exposure to sunlight for 25-30 minutes. An early study by Stamp confirmed vitamin D-3 supplementation was as effective as sun exposure. Further research shows oral vitamin D-3 (a by-product of sheep's wool or pigskin source) more effective than vitamin D-2 (yeast source). Therefore, we recommend a daily minimum of 4,000 IU of vitamin D-3 if you have an auto-immune illness such as MS. This 4,000 IU is equal to 0.1 mg, or 100 mcg and will cost you about 5 cents per day. Dr. Bill takes this year-round, despite sun exposure in our Canadian four-month summer window. Don't rely on your multivitamin to provide this amount of vitamin D, as multivitamins usually contain only 400-600 IU. Look for a separate vitamin D supplement that provides 1,000 IU per tablet. Vitamin D can now be purchased in a gel cap combined with olive oil. Because vitamin D is fat soluble, this would improve its absorption.

Vitamin D is now known to reduce the risk of at least 16 cancers including bowel, prostate, breast, and ovarian cancers. There is also strong evidence for vitamin D's role in preventing type 1 diabetes, and reduced levels of vitamin D induce insulin resistance, which is a risk for type 2 diabetes. Low levels of vitamin D have also been linked to obesity, high blood pressure, muscle weakness in the elderly, depression, inflammatory bowel disease, rheumatoid arthritis, and heart failure. In addition, vitamin D has a beneficial effect on our immune system in regards to healing infections, particularly tuberculosis and other auto-immune illnesses such as psoriasis.

Janet Raloff wrote a two-part series in *Science News* (www.science-news.org) in 2004 called "Vitamin D, What Is Enough?" Her summary of the story of vitamin D would at first appear simple. "Take in enough sun, or drink enough fortified milk to get the recommended daily amount, and you'll have strong bones. Take a supplement if you want insurance." But recent studies from around the world have revealed that the sunshine vitamin's role in health is far more complex. More than just protecting bone, vitamin D is proving to preserve muscle strength and to give some protection against deadly diseases including multiple sclerosis (MS), diabetes, and even cancer.

More like a Hormone

Vitamin D is more like a hormone than a vitamin. Bone-metabolism specialist, Robert P. Heaney, states that vitamin D is a misnomer: "A vitamin is an essential food constituent that the body can't make." He expands on this notion by explaining that we make vitamin D in our skin from a cholesterol-like precursor. Our body can generate 10,000-12,000 units (250-300 mcg) of vitamin D in 30 minutes of summer sunshine. And yet, most people in the United States get well below the recommended 200-600 IU/day, especially in winter. Americans living above Los Angeles, Canadians, and Northern Europeans are particularly in need of vitamin D supplementation because of the lack of effective sunshine for vitamin D production from October to April. We know from Canadian studies of blood vitamin D levels that adults have a blood level below 40 in winter months. This is far too low to reap the health benefits seen with higher blood levels of vitamin D. When we heed dermatologists' warning about preventing skin cancer by limiting sun exposure and using sunscreen, we also reduce our vitamin D production. At present, there is a visible lawsuit proceeding involving an early advocate of increased vitamin D. In Boston, Dr. M. F. Holick is suing to get his academic position back. It was "stripped" from him because his vitamin D position was too far outside the opinion of the major American scientific community. We are supporting Holick on this one!

Heike Bischoff-Ferrari, now at Harvard, measured vitamin D blood concentrations in elderly men and women. Individuals with higher readings also had greater thigh strength. Bischoff-Ferrari then launched an intervention trial with 122 women in their mid-80s. Everyone received 1,200 mg of calcium per day, and half received 800 IU of vitamin D.

After three months, each woman was tested for leg strength and how easily she could get up from a chair, walk around an object, and sit back down. Not only did the vitamin D–supplemented women perform dramatically better, but they also sustained only half as many falls. Falls, of course, are a leading cause of fracture and disability and are believed to cost $20 billion U.S. each year in medical bills.

WHO COULD BENEFIT FROM VITAMIN D SUPPLEMENTS?

1. *Pre-pregnant and pregnant women*
2. *Babies*
3. *Children*
4. *Adolescents*
5. *Adults*
6. *Seniors*
7. *Everyone—vitamin D inadequacy is widespread, especially for people living further from the equator and those limiting sun exposure.*

You can see clearly from this study that vitamin D supplementation is more than just "slowing down" or "reversing" osteoporosis. It is no longer just enough to have the long-recommended DRI, because this amount is only enough to prevent rickets. Rickets (bowed legs in children) is actually on the increase in Canada and the United Kingdom. Dark-skinned children are especially at risk, as they require more time in the sunshine to make the same amount of vitamin D.

In addition, careful studies of pregnancy and time of year of delivery reveal that those born in spring are more at risk of MS because the pregnant moms tend to have much less vitamin D in winter months. Better protection exists for babies born in late autumn due to the greater levels of vitamin D. Some nutrition experts are suggesting that vitamin D supplementation (we suggest at least 1,000 IU and feel 2,000 IU is even better) is as important in pregnancy as folic acid is.

ADEQUATE VITAMIN D:

- *prevents many types of cancer and outcome linked to vitamin D status—higher vitamin D linked to better outcome.*
- *reduces pain of major auto-immune illness*
- *prevents auto-immune diseases*
- *prevents osteoporosis*
- *reduces inflammatory pain*
- *helps depression*
- *improves muscle strength and balance*
- *helps fibromyalgia, osteoarthritis, and tuberculosis*
- *improves high blood pressure and heart failure*

Of course, the newborn child should immediately be on a vitamin supplement containing vitamin D. We know that 1,000 IU of vitamin D in a one-year-old infant and onward much reduces the child's risk of type 1 diabetes, MS, rheumatoid arthritis, and childhood cancers. In addition, there is considerable increased risk of MS in our own children, due to both Dr. Bill and a sister having been diagnosed with MS. If only in one parent, the risk is 2-3%; however, the risk more than doubles if a parent's sibling also has MS. The daily dose of vitamin D we are recommending—4,000 IU or 100 mcg— is very inexpensive, safe, and it serves as valuable health insurance.

Osteoporosis prevention has inclined many calcium product manufacturers to include vitamin D in the calcium supplement. However, this is only a small, very modest amount of vitamin D. Often this is 200 IU per 500 mg calcium. The vitamin D helps improve absorption of calcium from the gut from 20-30% up to 80%. Calcium is best absorbed with food and, ideally, only 500 mg of elemental calcium should be taken at one time. Larger doses of calcium are not as effectively absorbed.

Besides limited amounts of sunshine to produce adequate vitamin D in the body, we also have a problem getting enough vitamin D from food. Vitamin D sources include fish liver oils; fish such as salmon, mackerel, and sardines; and eggs. Small amounts of vitamin D are found in pork liver, beef liver, and butter. Health Canada realized years ago that, to prevent scurvy, supplemental vitamin D was needed. This led to vitamin fortification of fluid milk and of margarine. Milk contains 100 IU vitamin D per 250 ml; margarine contains 33 IU per tsp (5 ml). Remember, it is only milk that vitamin D is added to; cheese, yogurt, ice cream, and other dairy products are not fortified with vitamin D.

WHY MEASURE VITAMIN D?

1. *To obtain baseline blood levels or determine adequacy of vitamin D supplementation.*

2. *Physicians are overly concerned about toxicity of vitamin D supplementation.*

3. *Current lab values for normal blood vitamin D are too low for optimal health.*

4. *Toxicity levels are much higher than previously believed—500 nmol/l, not 140 nmol/l.*

5. *Blood levels greater than 120 nmol/l are needed for therapeutic benefit for chronic illness.*

6. *People vary in their absorption from vitamin D supplements so baseline vitamin D level should be measured before supplementation and follow-up every three months is recommended.*

Vitamin D and Pain

Supplementation with vitamin D can help prevent osteoporosis and slow the process of osteoporosis, secondary bone collapse, and consequent neuropathic pain. Thus, chronic pain sufferers should have noted that vitamin D has a role in pain prevention. In addition, vitamin D at 2,000 IU/day, or 0.05 mg, is now accepted as reducing inflammation. What concerns us about pain and inflammation? Remember that inflammation is by definition redness, swelling, heat, and pain or loss of function. Hence, Dr. Bill suggests that vitamin D supplementation is useful to both prevent pain and to reduce pain of inflammation, whatever the inflammatory trigger, as inflammation is the key step in our healing process.

What about the safety of doses of vitamin D-3 in the range of 1,000-4,000 IU daily? The recommended intake for adults has been set much lower: 200 IU for adults over age 20, 400 IU for adults 51-70, and 600 IU for adults over 70. Yet, much of the scientific literature points to a higher level of vitamin D for disease treatment and prevention. Vieth has written many articles and is emphatic that the "no observed adverse effect level (NOAEL) is at least 10,000 IU/day. He does state that levels of vitamin D of 40,000 IU/day would be a problem. Thus, a level of 4,000 IU/day is perfectly safe. Vieth stresses that his recommendations are for vitamin D-3 (cholecalciferol) not vitamin D-2 or other forms of vitamin D.

It is seven years now that Dr. Bill has been taking vitamin D at 4,000 IU or 100 mcg or 0.1 mg per day, year-round. His vitamin D is still only 99, which is considered optimal for helping minimize MS symptoms. We therefore suggest that you get with the program: sunshine plus supplementation, and if in doubt, have your blood vitamin D measured. Aim for more than 100 nmol/liter. Recent literature suggests up to 500 nmol/liter is quite safe.

CHAPTER SIX

Emu Oil: A Natural Anti-Inflammatory

W̲e believe that Dr. Bill's daily intake (1 tsp or 5 ml) of emu oil was the first dietary supplement that helped in his initial recovery from fatigue! That was a huge and positive shift from despair to hope! Oral emu oil seemed to enhance his energy, which was pitifully low for 12 or more months. As we thought about it, we came to believe emu oil's safe and natural anti-inflammatory effects were quite possibly the reasons for his enhanced well-being.

It is now accepted that our body uses inflammation as part of the healing process, regardless of the organ, tissue, or time of life. Our understanding from this premise is that a similar type of healing occurs in our brain. In those of us with illnesses involving demyelinating nerves (such as MS and Guillain Barre syndrome), neurons are injured by the white blood cells attacking their myelin sheath. During this process, free radicals are produced. The surrounding nerves, blood vessels, and glial cells (astrocytes) sustain injury from these free radicals. While the glutathione, a potent antioxidant, quenches the free radicals, the emu oil may play a part in fine-tuning the healing response in the brain just as it does on the skin. This fine-tuning may speed the healing process and, in addition, reduce the local scarring around the nerves.

Daily emu oil may provide this "injury reducing" anti-inflammatory effect whenever pain or an MS flare-up occurs. We think of it as a very safe, natural anti-inflammatory, perhaps reducing the need for cortisone steroid use when severe attacks occur. We also now have a strong aversion to steroids, even though at one time we advocated their use. We think that, whenever possible, people with MS, rheumatoid arthritis, systemic lupus, and many other chronic illnesses should avoid using oral or intravenous corticosteroids. This would include avoiding injections of steroids into joints and epidural steroids for low back pain and neck pain.

The Australian study by Snowden and Whitehouse (see *References*) showed that topical emu oil was more effective as an anti-inflammatory in wrist soreness and stiffness (arthritis) than a considerable dose of ibuprofen, a Non-Steroidal Anti-Inflammatory Drug (NSAID). Lopez and his research team (see *References*) also demonstrated that emu oil was anti-inflammatory in an inflamed skin model much like eczema. In addition, there has never been any suggestion that emu oil slowed healing, as NSAIDs do. To the contrary, emu oil doubles the rate of wound healing and quadruples it relative to cortisone in a skin model of research, studied by Politis (see *References*).

Despite 35 years of using corticosteroids (ACTH was an early form), doctors have never been able to prove or show that they have any lasting benefit to people with MS, lupus, or rheumatoid arthritis. In fact, just the opposite, physicians know that steroids can trigger occasional hip joint death, can create early or premature cataracts, and frequently can worsen osteoporosis. Hip joint death is sometimes triggered by a single dose of corticosteroids. Somehow, the drug shuts down or blocks the blood supply to the joint lining. Once it dies, joint replacement is inevitable. In all of Dr. Bill's years in medicine and now as a person with an auto-immune illness, rarely has he heard physicians say, "I have nothing to offer." If pushed, they will often fall back on corticosteroids, oral or intravenous. In all fairness, it is we patients who ask, "Can't you do something?!" If you have an acute MS flare-up, are blind, and/or paralyzed and have no help or assistance to care for young children, you may have no recourse but to use corticosteroids. As a general rule, though, avoid them whenever possible.

Emu oil provides three major benefits. The first is skin care, a particular concern in a dry, low-humidity climate such as Alberta, Canada, or Colorado in the United States. For people with post-herpetic neuralgia (pain after shingles), MS, or diabetes, reduced touch or skin sensation is common. This, plus dry, itchy skin, can be a poor combination. The moisturizing, penetration, and anti-inflammatory effects of pure emu oil or a cream thereof may delay or even avoid skin tears, burns, or pressure ulcers (bed sores) and even diabetic wounds or ulcers.

Second, emu oil has the ability to relieve pain, both externally and internally. The pain relief of emu oil may be found with topical application or oral capsules, or both. The most obvious example is shingles (herpes zoster, chicken pox, or varicella in children). Topical application of emu oil can eliminate the pain from shingles for up to two hours. A reapplication works for another two hours and so on. As expected, the blisters or scabs heal up faster. We believe this single therapy can reduce greatly the likelihood of severe, ongoing "neuropathic" pain of post-herpetic neuralgia. This pain syndrome afflicts at least 5% of shingles sufferers who respond poorly to oral medications. In fact, up to 5% of these people go on to commit suicide—the pain is so severe and all consuming. We believe this shingles neuropathic pain is similar to the neuropathic pain of MS. Seventy percent of people with MS seek prescription medication for pain. Even a 20-50% reduction in this pain could improve our quality of life. Yes, Dr. Bill routinely takes five 500 mg emu oil capsules per day orally as a safe anti-inflammatory with some pain-relief effect. (See *Appendix A & B*.)

BENEFITS OF EMU OIL

1. *Penetrates the skin safely, without toxicity.*

2. *Is anti-inflammatory—likely due to its carotenoids.*

3. *Provides pain relief for sore muscles and also for shingles and herpes simplex.*

4. *Speeds skin healing*

5. *Is non-comedogenic (does not clog pores) and does not cause acne.*

Dr. M. Holick, MD, PhD, Boston (mentioned in Chapter 5), wonderfully described emu oil's ability to make skin up to one-third thicker. In addition, he noted that it helps regrow the connecting "rete pegs" between our two skin layers—the epidermis and dermis. These two attributes of emu oil reduce, even help reverse, wrinkles and make us look and feel younger. Also, topical or oral emu oil wake up 35-40% of sleeping hair cells. Most of us, especially women, are delighted to regain thicker hair.

Thinning of our hair and loss of skin glow are commonly associated with poor health and/or chemotherapy. Chemotherapeutic drugs are used not just with cancer, but also in MS, psoriasis, rheumatoid arthritis, and lupus. Isn't it great to have an alternative such as emu oil, a natural product that is safe and can be used orally or topically?

Dr. Bill and his two sons use emu oil on their faces after shaving and when the climate is dry, in high-altitude locations, and of course on airplanes. Dr. Bill now considers emu oil as an option for most skin troubles including itching, pain, scaling, redness, swelling, or any such inflammation problems. We like making people's day with the gift of an emu oil—based lip balm. They usually become fans for good—especially if cold sores trouble them.

Similarly, when Dr. Bill has leg muscle spasms, he will apply a topical joint comfort mixture containing 20% emu oil plus glucosamine, methyl sulfonyl methane, boswellia, cetyl myristoleate (a fatty acid that assists soft tissue healing), devil's claw extract, and peppermint. (See *Appendix A & B*.) This mixture has helped many people with leg cramps and muscle spasms due to MS and works more often than Dr. Bill expected it to. The emu oil at 20% will have some direct benefits of its own and also acts as a carrier of other compounds through the skin. (A recent study confirmed emu oil's ability to carry vitamin E through the skin and to raise the concentration of vitamin E in the blood.)

People suffering from arthritis pain, muscle cramps, or stiff joints will be delighted with the joint comfort mentioned above. (See *Appendix A & B*.) It should be applied once or twice daily, as required. Dr. Bill's dad loved it

for his leg cramps at night; it helped him go right back to sleep. Dr. Bill especially likes this product, as the emu oil and other natural components it
carries deep through the skin act synergistically (well together) to promote
soft tissue healing. This is very much unlike the NSAIDs and cortisone,
which retard healing of skin, ligaments, tendons, cartilage, and bone.

A second pain relief product Dr. Bill likes is an oily rub combining
mainly emu oil with wintergreen, eucalyptus, and camphor for pain that is
resistant to the joint comfort mentioned above. The wintergreen acts as aspirin,
so this would best be avoided in people on warfarin (Coumadin), the blood
thinner drug. However, if joint comfort cream and this emu oil/wintergreen
combination are both used, the pain relief is tremendous.

Finally, we want to thank the emu oil and the emu bird for important
components of Dr. Bill's healing journey with chronic pain, dry, thinning
hair, and muscle spasms. Our small acreage on Vancouver Island, off the
West Coast, provided a healing milieu. Prominent in this was the emu life
cycle, the beauty and peace of nature, and the gift of the ability to look
within for mind and spiritual issues. This wonderful environment, combined
with the increasing awareness of body, mind, and spiritual interaction, initiated some real recovery for Dr. Bill's chronic pain, muscle spasms, fatigue,
and stiffness. Most auto-immune pain, arthritis pain, chronic fatigue pain,
and fibromyalgia pain can benefit considerably as well.

CHAPTER SEVEN

Dietary Fat: The Good and the Bad

Our brain is 60% fat, so the next time you are called a "fathead" take it as a compliment. Omega-3 fatty acids are by far the most important fats for brain development, function, healing, and recovery. There are two essential fatty acids (EFAs) that we need. Omega-6 includes linoleic acid, gamma linolenic acid (GLA), and arachidonic acid (not to be confused with arachidic acid, which is from peanuts). Omega-3, now thought to be the most essential fatty acid, is without a doubt the most important for our brains. The omega-3 family includes alpha-linolenic acid, EPA, and DHA (see Figure 1.1). We will list sources, especially of omega-3, because almost everyone in North America is deficient in this one. For the record, for optimal health, the intake of saturated fats must be moderate and trans fats near zero.

EFAs Made Simple

EFAs play a role in every cell in the body. Their curved shape—like curves in a caterpillar—are absolutely critical for making healthy body cells, including brain cells called neurons and glia (astrocytes). If either omega-6 or omega-3 oils are hydrogenated, they become trans fatty acids.[1] Trans fats tend to be straight, and they greatly reduce the normal health and function of every cell, including brain cells. North Americans have had trans fats from hydrogenated oils in our diet for over 50 years.

---

[1] Hydrogenation is a process that converts a liquid oil to a solid fat. In this process, heat and hydrogen gas are added to the liquid oil. The chemical reaction that occurs adds hydrogen atoms to the oil and the oil becomes solid.

Shortening, hard margarine, baked goods, and deep-frying oils (e.g., for frying potato chips) all contain trans fats. You must learn to read labels, for your own protection and long-term health. Remember, all our body's cells are gradually changed and replaced over time. Hence, healing is possible even in the brain and spinal cord.

We routinely read food labels, even those on chocolate bars, in order to avoid all "modified," "hydrogenated," or "trans" fats. All of these names denote trans fats. Identification gets easier all the time, as awareness

---

Fatty Acids Made Simple

The Omega-6 Family	**The Omega-3 Family**
Linoleic Acid (LA)	Alpha-Linolenic Acid (ALA)
(LA is found in vegetable oils, seeds, and nuts.)	(ALA is found in green leafy vegetables, flax, flaxseed oil, hemp oil, canola oil, emu oil, walnuts, and Brazil nuts.)
Your body converts LA into:	Your body converts ALA into:
↓	↓
Gamma-Linolenic Acid (GLA)	Eicosapentaenoic Acid (EPA)
(GLA is also found in borage and primrose oil.)	(EPA is also found in fish oil.)
Your body converts GLA into:	Your body converts EPA into:
↓	↓
Arachidonic Acid (AA)	Docosahexaenoic Acid (DHA)
(AA is also found in meat.)	(DHA is also found in fish oil.)
↓	↓
The Omega-6 Family of Eicosanoids Unhappy or Inflammatory Prostaglandins	The Omega-3 Family of Eicosanoids Happy or Anti-Inflammatory Prostaglandins

Figure 1.1 Adapted from: The Omega Diet *by A. Simopoulos, M.D. & J. Robinson, Harper Perennial, 1999, p. 40*

increases. In fact, manufacturers are now using "No Trans Fats" as a marketing tool. This is a great help. Similarly, we do not order restaurant or take-out food that has been deep-fried or that has had trans fats used in its baking process. Pay attention to the choices of your salad dressings, too. If you are in doubt use olive oil, high in monounsaturated fats. Saturated fats, in moderation only, are much safer than trans fats. For cooking we use butter, but if high heat is needed (e.g., deep-frying), we recommend coconut, peanut, or palm oil.

More and more evidence is emerging that trans fats aggravate pain issues by worsening cellular inflammation. Inflammation, which as you know by now is pain (loss of function), redness, swelling, and heat, is promoted or worsened at the cellular level. On April 13, 2006, an article in the *New England Journal of Medicine (NEJM)* reviewed the latest evidence concerning the presence of trans fats in the American diet and the negative impact of trans fats on human health. This article, jointly submitted by the Harvard Medical School, the Harvard School of Public Health, and others, concludes that "complete or near avoidance of trans fats ... may be necessary to avoid adverse risks." One of these adverse risks is pain and flare-up of a chronic disease having inflammatory pain associated with it. This major review article suggests less than 0.5% of total energy intake be trans fats.

BENEFITS OF REDUCING BAD FATS (ESPECIALLY TRANS FATS)

1. *Less atherosclerosis (heart disease and strokes)*
2. *More optimal cell function*
3. *Less inflammatory pain*
4. *Healthier brain cells and better brain function*
5. *Improved healing of all cells, including brain cells*

A 2004 article in *American Journal of Clinical Nutrition* by Mozaffarian showed an important link between trans fatty acids and systemic inflammation in women. These researchers and others also from the Harvard School of Public Health have sounded the alarm about trans fats since the early 1990s. Recently the FDA in the United States ruled that the amount of trans fat must be included on the label. This change is causing a makeover of the American food supply. The FDA once estimated that 95% of prepared cookies, 100% of crackers, and 80% of frozen breakfast products contained trans fat. Trans fat is also found in fast foods. For example, a large order of fries at McDonald's delivers 6 grams of trans fat. Yet, in trans-free Denmark, McDonald's produces fries that are trans free! More and more products advertised as trans fat free are appearing on the shelves in the supermarkets. However, do not be lulled into thinking that these are necessarily healthier for you. Many of them still contain lots of fat and calories. Be sure to read the labels so that you know what you are buying (and eating)!

WHY REDUCE OMEGA-6 FATS?

1. *Contribute to inflammation in the body*

2. *Compete for enzymes in the omega-3 pathway and interfere with the production of omega-3 EPA and DHA*

3. *Intake of oils high in omega-6 replaces intake of healthier omega-3 fats*

Our hope is that you now understand that trans fats are the very bad fats. Saturated fats and liquid oils, if used in moderation, are the very good fats. Liquid oils contain monounsaturated (MUFA)[2] and polyunsaturated (PUFA) fat, which are generally considered as healthy fats. However, we want to specify which PUFAs are most important to people with MS or to those who have other inflammations, including ALS, fibromyalgia, arthritis (osteo, rheumatoid), psoriasis, asthma, Meniere's, Parkinson's, lupus, chronic fatigue syndrome, and all other inflammatory conditions. In fact, it is now thought that inflammation occurs in every disease process. In short, avoid or minimize oils very high in omega-6 fatty acids. This would include corn, safflower, grapeseed, sunflower, and soybean oils.

---

[2] Fat contains long chains of carbon atoms. Attached to the carbon atoms are oxygen and hydrogen. When a fat holds all the hydrogen that it can, it is called a saturated fat. Butter, lard and coconut oil are all saturated. They are also solid fats. If a fat has room for one more hydrogen, it is monounsaturated. Olive oil, canola oil and peanut oil are monounsaturated fats (MUFAs) and are liquid. If a fat has room for 2 or more hydrogen atoms, they are polyunsaturated fats. Corn oil and safflower oils are polyunsaturated fats (PUFAs) and liquid.

Please refer to the omega-6 and omega-3 pathways diagram (Figure 1.1), and note that each pathway has a Family of Eicosanoids (or prostaglandins) at the bottom. These are designed to counterbalance one another. Also, remember, almost all of the unhappy or unpleasant prostaglandins are at the end of the omega-6 pathway. These trigger the inflammation associated with arthritis, asthma, menstrual cramps, hay fever (allergic rhinitis), the swelling of the nerves in MS, or the joint inflammation in arthritis attacks, and the inflammation associated with degenerative diseases.

Composition of Selected Fats (by %)*

Oil or Fat	Omega-3 %	Omega-6 %	Oleic Acid %	Saturated Fat %
Lard (pig)	0.01	6.7	39.4	48.1
Tallow (beef)	1.5	2.3	43.1	40.6
Ostrich	1.9	16.0	30.5	40.0
Emu	1.7	16.0	53.0	29.0
Chicken Fat	1.0	20.0	45.0	30.0
Olive	0.0	8.0	82.0	10.0
Flax	57.0	18.0	16.0	9.0
Canola	10.0	24.0	60.0	6.0
Soybean	7.0	58.0	23.0	14.0
Peanuts	0.0	31.7	49.3	13.8
Corn	0.0	59.0	24.0	12.0
Sunflower	0.0	66.0	20.0	10.0
Cottonseed	1.0	40.0	18.0	31.0
Safflower	0.4	75.0	12.0	9.0
Grapeseed	0.0	70.0	16.0	10.0
Borage	0.0	78.0	0.0	0.0
Primrose	0.0	81.0	11.0	8.0
Walnuts	10.0	53.0	23.0	9.0
Almonds	0.01	20.1	65.1	9.6
Brazil Nuts	0.0	36.0	34.6	24.3

*There are monounsaturates other than oleic, so total fats may not add up to 100%.

Omega-3 Oils Rule

Unfortunately, at least 80% of North Americans have much more omega-6 in our diet than omega-3. We consume nearly 20 times more omega-6 fats than omega-3 fats. Consequently, we suffer from an excess of the omega-6 "unhappy" eicosanoids or prostaglandins. Why? We are victims of our own shopping preferences. We have a huge selection of processed and packaged foods in our grocery stores—crackers, cookies, cake mixes, sauces, dips, baked goods, and more. These usually contain vegetable oils high in omega-6 fat. Furthermore, these vegetable oils have been modified or hydrogenated, resulting in harmful trans fats.

We expect any product to be odorless, or at least not to smell rancid; hence the rampant marketing and sales of not only trans fats, but also of oils high in omega-6 fatty acids, as omega-6 oils keep much better on the store shelf than do omega-3 oils. Omega-3 fatty acids easily break down and become rancid. This explains the relative unpopularity of taking a spoonful of cod liver oil and many fish oils—they can have a strong odor and flavor.

What about the long-touted evening primrose oil, or more recent borage oil, for multiple sclerosis and other illnesses? Despite three decades of studies testing these in MS, we have no confirming studies of note. We will suggest a reason for this conundrum. Evening primrose oil and borage oil contain GLA, which belongs to the omega-6 family. Converting linoleic acid (omega-6) to GLA and alpha-linolenic acid (omega-3) to EPA requires the same enzyme. (See Figure 1.1). By adding more GLA, less of the enzyme is needed for converting linoleic acid to GLA. This leaves more of the enzyme available for converting alpha-linolenic acid to EPA and DHA, two key brain fats. However, most people's diets are very low in alpha-linolenic acid. Therefore, only a small amount of alpha-linolenic can be converted to EPA and the benefits would be minimal.

GLA supplementation is generally not advised. According to Franco Cavaleri, GLA supplementation can "fuel more disease if unhealthy dietary habits aren't changed at the same time." GLA can be converted to arachidonic acid in the cells. Arachidonic acid can then be transformed into prostaglandins that promote inflammation. As mentioned previously, many of our diseases also have inflammation associated with them. Therefore, we would not want to add to the inflammation process by increasing GLA. It is recommended that anyone supplementing with borage oil or evening primrose oil should also take a fish oil supplement. This will reduce arachidonic acid production and subsequent inflammation.

A wealth of studies support the health benefits of omega-3 fats. They play an important role in brain health, heart health, skin health, immune function, joint mobility, and protection against inflammation and cancer. The omega-3 parent, alpha-linolenic acid, is found in plant sources. The richest sources are flax, hemp, canola, soybean, and walnut. The alpha-linolenic acid can then be converted to EPA and DHA. Fish oil is a rich source of EPA and DHA.

Unfortunately, the conversion of alpha-linolenic acid to DHA is limited. Much of the dietary alpha-linolenic acid is oxidized and, on average, only 3.8% becomes EPA that is then converted to DHA. In addition, a deficiency in zinc, magnesium, vitamin C, vitamin B-3, or vitamin B-6 will impair conversion to EPA and production of the "happy" prostaglandins. Because our diets contain so little alpha-linolenic acid, and limited EPA is produced from it, a more efficient way to get EPA and DHA is from fish oil supplements. Indeed, research has shown that EPA increases more in body cells when a fish oil supplement is given with dietary alpha-linolenic acid.

The use of fish oils and the fact that they contain high amounts of EPA and DHA merits special mention. EPA and DHA are particularly important in the first year of human life for ongoing brain development. EPA and DHA are essential at this time, and breast milk is still considered the best source. The mother can enhance the amount of omega-3s in her breast milk by taking a good omega-3 supplement. Similarly, infant formulas should have the omega-3 oils added to them. In most countries, this has already occurred. In Canada, DHA has just recently been added to infant formula.

More recently, krill oil has become available as a supplement. Krill oil comes from a tiny shrimp-like creature that is an important food source for whales, penguins, and fish. Krill oil is rich in EPA and DHA and has powerful antioxidants such as vitamin A, vitamin E, and astaxathin. The antioxidant activity in krill oil is 550 times more potent than vitamin E alone. The ratio of omega-3 to omega-6 is extremely high: 30:1. Furthermore, krill oil has a high level of phospholipids, which are vital to brain function, spinal cord, and nerves. Most fish oils do not provide these phospholipids. Krill oil not only provides unique brain health benefits, but also a more concentrated amount of EPA and DHA.

Two potential downsides of fish and fish oils are their cost and the toxins they carry. In recent recommendations, most of us should eat canned tuna only once a week—due to the heavy metals, dioxins, and other contaminants in the tuna. Similarly, farmed salmon can contain significant levels of toxins depending on the location it is farmed and the type of feed and origin of the feed. For example, salmon originating from the North Sea (above Europe) has a reasonably high toxic load. It is generally thought that the benefits of DHA and EPA from eating fish far outweigh the risks associated with contaminants, including methyl mercury. Eating fish several times per week is certainly one way to get your DHA and EPA. If you prefer to minimize your toxic load, then limit your fish consumption and use pharmaceutical grade fish oil supplements. These are only recommendations and will vary according to your use of safe, healthy detoxification choices—namely taking glutathione-building blocks of bioactive cysteine and/or infrared sauna with sand emitter in the 6-20 micron range.

Toxicity and taste issues of fish oils can be overcome by purchasing fish oils that have undergone a purification process. Ensure that you buy quality, pharmaceutical-grade fish oils. Increased cost is the downside. Always keep in mind that cold-water fish is higher in the healthy omega-3 fats than warm-water fish. Similarly, krill oil has a high level of omega-3s and is perhaps superior to fish oil because it has a higher level of DHA and also contains beneficial phospholipids for brain health. The downside of krill oil is that it is expensive.

Flax Is a Great Solution, Plus Fish Oils

For a host of reasons, we strongly recommend flax as a source of omega-3s. First, it is safe, as it has no fish-related heavy metals and dioxins, and second, it is the least expensive source of omega-3 fat. One to two tablespoons of ground flax seed provides 1.8-3.6 g alpha-linolenic acid. This meets the adequate intake of alpha-linolenic acid for adults. Third, ground flax is 25% soluble and 75% insoluble fiber. This high fiber content has a great "brush, brush" cleansing ability within our large bowel. In addition, the fiber absorbs toxins from the bowel, including those excreted in the bile. For example, drug reabsorption is lowered, as are heavy metals and the "bad" cholesterol—Low Density Lipoprotein, or LDL. Fourth, flax's rich brown seed-coat contains lignans, which reduce our risk of bowel cancer, breast cancer, prostate cancer, heart attack, and stroke. Considering the three leading causes of death in North America are heart disease, cancer, and stroke, respectively, we should take advantage of all these benefits of flax. The fiber is also a useful asset to many of us with MS, as we tend toward constipation.

An important side note here is that flax is acceptable to people with celiac disease. For those who are truly allergic to flax, the next best option is ground hemp or hemp oil. Allergic reactions to both hemp and flax are fortunately quite uncommon. Hemp is a two-to-one ratio of omega-6 to omega-3 and also has a reasonable amount of GLA. This is good news for those who are already using GLA and who would rather "fight than switch." (Remember, though, to also take a fish oil supplement.)

An easy option is to eat 2-3 tablespoons of ground flax (30-45 ml) every day. It can be added to hot cereal (oatmeal), cold cereal, salads, muffins, breads (made with grains you *can* tolerate), or even spread on toast. Whole flax seed keeps well for many months. Once flax is ground in a coffee grinder or kitchen blender, it keeps well for several weeks. We usually grind enough for a week to 10 days and then store it in a cool place. Refrigeration is fine, but not necessary. Make sure you add flax to your diet daily, as a habit. Even though people often say, "You must use it in the next 20-30 minutes after grinding," we find this advice a bit "over the top." It will not lose its freshness that quickly. For those who can not or choose not to have ground flax, flax oil is an option. However, it will not have the fiber and lignan advantages of ground flax. Flax oil comes in bottles or capsules and must be stored in the refrigerator to prevent it from going rancid.

WHY MORE FLAX, KRILL, AND FISH OILS?

1. *Better brain health*

2. *Reduce chronic pain and neuropathic pain*

3. *Reduce inflammation from omega-6 oils*

4. *Reduce depression*

5. *Reduce heart attacks and strokes*

6. *Improve the body's ability to make "happy" anti-inflammatory prostaglandins*

For post-menopausal women having hot flashes or "power surges," flax has significant phytoestrogens. These are equivalent to soy phytoestrogens and are an excellent alternative for those concerned about excess soy in the diet. Another important issue to address is the "cyano" or cyanide factor with flax. This is no problem whatsoever and is well addressed in the superb book on flax *Flaxseed in Human Nutrition*. Expert, J. K. Daun informs us that when the cyanide equivalent is calculated in, an adult can consume more than one kilogram (2.2 lb) per day before exhibiting acute cyanic toxicity.

In summary, ground flax intake of 30-45 ml (2-3 tbs.) per day is very high on Dr. Bill's "Top 10 Supplement Choices" list. Flax grown in cool areas such as Northern Europe, South Australia, or Western Canada is the highest in polyunsaturated fatty acids. Ensure adequate amounts of EPA and DHA by eating fish and taking fish oil supplements. A combination of all three—flax, fish, and purified fish oils—will help you meet your omega-3 needs.

Omega-3s for Pain

A very interesting article on omega-3 fatty acids (fish oil) as an anti-inflammatory was published by J. C. Maroon and J. W. Bost, researchers from the Department of Neurological Surgery, University of Pittsburgh Medical Center, who studied omega-3s versus nonsteroidal anti-inflammatory drugs (NSAIDs) for discogenic pain. The neurosurgeons gave 250 patients questionnaires to complete. Of the 250 patients, 125 returned the questionnaire. Seventy-eight percent of the patients were taking 1,200 mg of omega-3 oil and 22% were taking 2,400 mg of omega-3 oil. Of these, 59% quit taking their prescription NSAID medication for pain and 60% said their joint pain had improved. Eighty percent stated they were satisfied with their improvement and 88% said they would continue to take their fish oil. No significant side effects were reported. The authors stated that omega-3 essential fatty acids (fish oil) supplements appear to be a safer alternative to NSAIDs for treatment of non-surgical neck or back pain.

The optimal amount of omega-3 for health is still being investigated. Health Canada recommends 1.6 g/day alpha-linolenic acid for adult men and 1.1 g/day for adult women. Studies have shown that 900 mg/day of fish oil has a positive impact on mortality rates in patients with heart disease. This amount of fish oil can be obtained from eating salmon five times per week, or herring three times per week. A standard fish oil supplement provides 300 mg omega-3 fat per capsule.

Dr. Bruce Holub from the University of Guelph, Ontario, is one of Canada's leading experts on essential fatty acids. Through his research, he recommends the following amounts of omega-3 fatty acids: 300 mg/day for pregnant and breastfeeding women, 650 mg/day for healthy adults, and 900-1,000 mg/day for people with heart disease.

The evidence for the value of eliminating trans fats, reducing omega-6 fats, and increasing omega-3 fats is overwhelming. Evaluate the fats in your diet. Then make the necessary changes so that your diet includes the healthy fats every day. This will be a big, positive step in your health journey!

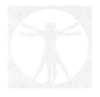

CHAPTER EIGHT

A Few of Our Favorite Things

We have structured this chapter to include helpful hints and tips for enhancing your coping skills and increasing your happiness while controlling your multiple sclerosis or other chronic illness. Many of these suggestions will add a great deal of joy to your life as well.

Natural Stress Management

Stress is a huge issue and we want to begin by mentioning a completely natural dietary supplement that helps the body resist or reduce stress. This supplement is a tiny protein (peptide) having a 10 amino acid ring. (See *Appendix A & B*.) This natural product was first patented in France and is now available in many countries worldwide including Canada, the United States, Australia, and many Asian countries. It is a peptide derived from milk and acts on the GABA receptor in the brain—the same receptor that works with valerian or the benzodiazepine drugs such as Valium, Serax, Ativan, and Librium. This peptide, like the drugs mentioned, relieves anxiety. Happily, this milk compound is non-addicting, does not suppress dream sleep (REM), and does not worsen our pain tolerance. All of the benzodiazepines have these disadvantages and, hence, are best avoided in MS and most other brain injuries or illnesses. For those wanting to reduce benzodiazepine use, please refer to *Point of Return,* which Dr. Bill co-authored with Alessandra Rain and Andrea Crocker, listed in *Appendix A & B.*

One to three capsules of this food, or nutraceutical, can reduce anxiety and help improve sleep. It can also lower cortisol, which is important in reducing abdominal fat. When the body is stressed, cortisol levels are high and the body tends to store food as fat.

Melatonin is another dietary supplement readily available in the United States and some other countries. Our body makes melatonin adequately on its own as long as two guidelines are followed. First, we have better quality sleep and produce more melatonin if we are in a totally dark room. Second, we need at least 15-20 minutes of bright, full-spectrum light per day to stimulate melatonin production in our body. One option is to purchase a "Seasonal Affective Disorder" (SAD) light and spend 15-20 minutes in front of it daily. Exposure to sunlight on a bright or sunny day will do this equally well. In fact, studies have documented that people working by a window have 7% improved productivity. However, some of us live in quite cloudy areas or are unable to get outside during the day or sit near a sunny window. An inexpensive alternative to using a SAD light is to get a full-spectrum light (usually fluorescent light, like those used to grow plants) and sit under it for 2-3 hours a day. We have seen this help a number of folks on the West Coast of Canada and the United States. (See *Appendix A & B*.) As you might expect from reading this far, we prefer to let our body produce melatonin with as little drug or supplement as possible. But, you decide what is best for you. It is your journey, not anyone else's!

WHY MORE MELATONIN?

1. *Reduces depression*
2. *Natural antioxidant, especially for the brain*
3. *Improved quality of sleep*

If you feel you need added help with stress management and sleep, try taking tart Montmorency cherry juice concentrate. This juice is naturally high in melatonin. An ounce of this concentrated juice prior to bedtime, diluted in 8 oz. (250 ml) of water, is very helpful. A further benefit to you may be the anti-inflammatory response of this tart extract. Friends have told us it is great for the pain of gouty arthritis. Similarly, it may be useful to use in conjunction with emu oil capsules or pain creams for the pain of inflamed muscles, tendons, ligaments, or joints.

Solution for Energy, Brain Fog, and Migraines

Our favorite energy drink is an herbal tonic that contains ginseng, gingko biloba, chamomile, damiana, angelica, and other herbs. (See *Appendix A & B*.) It also contains guarana—the most popular soft drink additive in Brazil. Research on guarana reveals its long use by the native people of the Amazon rain forest. Evidence suggests its use for relieving fatigue, boosting energy, aiding concentration, and brightening mood.

Guarana contains guaranine, a chemical substance with effects similar to caffeine. Yet, a dose of this tonic is equal to only 100 mg of caffeine, which is less than that in one cup of regular coffee. Even better, guarana gives 6-8 hours of slow burn, without the classic roller-coaster effects that many of us experience with coffee, tea, or cola drinks. If, like us, you feel jangled after drinking something with caffeine, you might want to consider this to reduce your caffeine intake or as a "brain fog" remedy.

Dr. Bill takes one ounce (30 ml) of this tonic every day. It immediately helps to boost potassium and magnesium in the body, and these increase alertness. Some people use this tonic twice a day. However, many of us will prefer to limit ourselves to one drink a day, to minimize side effects, such as diarrhea or stomach upset. Dr. Bill uses this early in the day, before 3:00 p.m., so that he can sleep fine at night. He also usually takes a half dose (15 ml) before exercising, as it improves stamina and he gets a better workout. Although the tonic is best taken early in the day, he often takes another dose at a later time, even at night, to "break" or stop a migraine. By the way, 80% of people with MS suffer migraines. The first line of defense against them is to avoid the foods to which you are sensitive. (Often it is wheat, wheat flour, and wheat pasta.)

Constipation Solutions

With constipation, prevention is number one. There is no such thing as "too much fiber." Ground flax is our all-time favorite, but psyllium, whole grains, and beans help too! Magnesium with calcium can be an effective option. If cost is a huge issue, take 0.5 teaspoon or 2.5 ml of magnesium sulfate (Epsom salts) in a glass of water, by mouth, and stay near a washroom or toilet. Plenty of good water, daily, is still very useful. Insist on eight glasses a day (250 ml or 8 oz. each) and aim for twelve!

Warm Mineral Baths for Muscle Relaxation

Before bed try a warm bath with bath salts, including a handful of magnesium sulfate (Epsom salts), as this will have several benefits. It will relax you and your muscles and perhaps even the sensors in your peripheral nerves. Hopefully, this will minimize the dreaded pains and muscle spasms so common with MS and other illnesses, especially during the night. We "discovered" the value of Epsom-salt baths from Dr. Bill's European-trained massage therapist, Isabella, prior to his two-day bicycle event for MS called the "Grape Escape" (see www.drbillcode.com for links to this MS Canada event on Vancouver Island, B.C.). Riding in this event also increased his enthusiasm for the energy drink; after four hours of cycling it reduced his groin muscle spasm and enabled him to lift his leg easily over the bicycle seat to mount and dismount!

Digestive Enzymes

Please do not interpret this next solution as just for "old people." By the age of 40, most of us experience reduced stomach acid secretion. This reduction in acid decreases the pre-digestion of our food. In addition, production of our regular enzymes (gallbladder, bile, and pancreas) declines. The end result is that our ability to recover nutrients from food is impaired. Therefore, reasonable use of digestive enzymes will allow us to digest and absorb nutrients more effectively from whole foods and to minimize other gastrointestinal symptoms. A good digestive enzyme will include lactase (acts on sugar in milk), lipase (acts on fat), and protease (acts on protein). Some enzymes also contain betaine hydrochloride to increase stomach acid. Enhanced digestion can decrease or eliminate heartburn, gas (burps or farts, too!), diarrhea, and constipation, and should maximize nutrient absorption from our diet. We much prefer the plant digestive enzymes to drugs for heartburn, as drugs reduce or even eliminate acid secretion, which then markedly reduces our normal digestive ability. See *Appendix A & B* for more choices of digestive enzymes.

Chocolate—Especially Dark Chocolate

Chocolate is a "mood elevator." For some of us, this is a sign that we need to "top up" our emotional energy and/or "slow down." Dark chocolate is "the best," hands down! It is full of beneficial antioxidants. But remember, read the labels to avoid those harmful trans (hydrogenated or modified) fats. Butter, palm oil, or coconut oil, in moderation, are better for health. Beware of the calories in chocolate: fat provides 9 calories per gram, as opposed to 4 calories per gram for protein and for carbohydrates. Also, watch out for liqueur chocolates: alcohol provides 7 calories per gram, and many of these chocolates are especially sweet. Use chocolate as an occasional treat. Weight gain tends to be a problem with people as they age. This can be even more of a problem for people who are not very active or who have physical limitations because of chronic pain, MS, or other health challenges.

WHY TAKE DIGESTIVE ENZYMES?

1. *Enzymes naturally produced in the body decline after age 40*
2. *Minimize heartburn*
3. *Better assimilation of nutrients from food*
4. *Reduce diarrhea, cramps and flatus (gas)*

Probiotics and Prebiotics

Our gut contains about 1-2 kilograms of friendly bacteria. These beneficial bacteria, such as Lactobacillus acidophilus and Bifidobacterium bifidum, are known as probiotics. These bacteria produce substances that promote the health of the cells lining the bowel. Too, these bacteria influence our general health. They inhibit the growth of harmful bacteria, increase our resistance to infection, and aid the immune system.

Traditionally, yogurt and fermented foods have been used for hundreds, if not thousands, of years to supply our bodies with probiotic bacteria. People eating a poor diet or suffering from diarrhea can be deficient in probiotic bacteria. Some drugs, especially antibiotics and some hormones, upset this natural process. A minimum use of probiotics would be advisable with hormone therapy such as estrogen (e.g., oral contraceptive or hormone replacement therapy) and drugs such as cortisone. People are advised to take probiotics following antibiotics in order to re-populate the gut with friendly bacteria.

A daily source of probiotics from food or supplements is recommended. This can be especially important while traveling and being exposed to different bacteria in food or the environment. In addition, minimize eating food that causes diarrhea or loose stools. This is important because the beneficial bacteria can be flushed out of the body. For many, the foods to avoid include fat, milk, lactose, legumes, beans, and beer because they all promote gastric hurry. Scientists claim that the food or probiotic supplement should supply from 1 million to 1 billion live bacteria in order to be effective. See *Appendix A & B* for probiotic choices.

Prebiotics are "food" for the friendly bacteria, to optimize their healthy synergy with us. These include fructo-oligosaccarides such as inulin, which cannot be digested or absorbed by humans, and are most useful if you are having trouble recovering from almost any bowel upset, including irritable bowel syndrome (IBS), a viral or gastrointestinal infection, dysentery, diverticulitis, bowel polyps, or if you are preparing for bowel surgery or radiology.

Calcium and Magnesium

Calcium, zinc, manganese, boron, and vitamin K are all important to slow down or even reverse osteoporosis. Therefore, build your calcium intake on a good multivitamin/multi-mineral base. Take at least half as much magnesium per day as calcium. We have found the easiest calcium to absorb is that derived from milk in the form of calcium phosphate. (See *Appendix A & B*.) Next-best sources of calcium are calcium citrate and calcium lactate. Dr. Bill currently aims for 2,000 mg/day of elemental calcium. Absorption is best when timed with food, in 500 mg per meal or snack, as acidity improves absorption, especially of calcium carbonate. Any of us, especially those of us with MS, who are not mobile or physically active are sitting ducks for osteoporosis. We suggest you get evaluated for bone density and be proactive against osteoporosis. Mobility is a further benefit because it will slow down your osteoporosis as well. Please remember, any corticosteroid use speeds up osteoporosis. So, think about the effects on your bones before you decide to take corticosteroids.

Cal/Emu

Twenty-five percent of North American adults over age 55 have knee pain. Cal/Emu is a new product combining type 2 collagen, calcium phosphorus, and magnesium—all of marine origin—plus emu oil in a gelatin capsule. The distinct value of type 2 collagen is well discussed in a review presentation by Kristine Clark, PhD, RD, Director of Sports Nutrition for Pennsylvania State University. Dr. Clark presented at the Nutrition for Joint Health 2003 World Congress. She cites eleven research articles on osteoarthritis confirming that this particular form of type 2 collagen reduces the pain and improves the mobility of those troubled with osteoarthritis. The research confirms absorption of this small molecule by the gut. In addition, the quality and quantity of cartilage is improved by the increased availability of this important cartilage building block. We know healthy collagen is dependent on adequate availability of calcium, vitamin D, phosphorus, vitamin C, and zinc. Those items not in this Cal/Emu combination are well covered by following Dr. Bill's "Top 10 Supplement Choices" for optimal health. See *Appendix A & B* at the end of the book for more information.

Infrared Sauna

We believe in infrared saunas, as mentioned earlier, but urge you to begin slowly. Start at the lower temperatures and only try it for 10-15 minutes every second day. If you do more, you might have more low energy days or poor-quality brain-thinking. The benefits of reducing toxins, probably enhanced cardiac fitness, and even weight loss while sitting on your butt will be worth the slow start-up!

Music

We think music has vast therapeutic effects contributing to relaxation, stress reduction, training backup brain pathways, and even improving breathing control and speech for the long term. We have enjoyed Dr. Bill's learning to play the Irish harp and eventually sing along with it. It has enhanced finger dexterity and also optimized the forming of new motor pathways. Singing is a great hobby, best done if you are rested, focused, and feeling well emotionally.

Future endeavors we recommend:

1) Horseback riding: This can be Western, English, or Therapeutic style. We love Winston Churchill's quote, "Time spent with a horse is never wasted."

2) Time spent with a dog: We believe this is both man and woman's best friend, as our dog will always forgive us.

3) Dance: Watch the movie *Shall We Dance* for inspiration, then get to know yourself and your partner better!

Dr. Bill's Top 10 Supplement Choices for Reversing Aging, Reducing Pain, and Improving Energy and Brain Function

1. **Undenatured whey protein isolate** – This optimizes the immune system, provides antioxidant benefits, and helps in detoxification. Quantity will depend on individual health needs.

2. **Daily omega-3 fat intake** – A daily fish oil supplement containing fish and/or krill oils is the best way to boost the omega-3 fat, especially EPA and DHA, needed for brain health. **Daily flax intake of 2-4 tablespoons of freshly ground brown flax** will supply alpha-linolenic acid (omega-3) fat and lignans. Lignans decrease the incidence of heart attack, stroke, and breast and colon cancer. Flax will also increase fiber intake for bowel health. Omega-3s will greatly reduce your risk of heart attack and stroke and pain due to inflammation.

3. **4,000 IU of vitamin D daily** – This will optimize the immune system, decrease the pain of inflammation, and reduce cancer and auto-immune conditions. This will also help your body absorb more calcium—important for preventing osteoporosis.

4. **One multivitamin/multi-mineral supplement daily** – Make sure it contains folic acid, B-6, and B-12. Tablets should disintegrate in water within two to four hours.

5. **Use of digestive enzymes (with each meal) and daily probiotics** – This will help enhance digestion and nutrient absorption.

6. **1,000 mg elemental calcium and 500 mg magnesium daily** – This will help maintain bone health and may reduce nerve irritability.

7. **Tart Montmorency cherry concentrate, 1 oz. (2 tbsp.) daily** – This is a potent source of antioxidants and an excellent source of anthocyanins, melatonin, and potassium.

8. **Emu oil daily** – Four to five gel caps will improve energy and mental focus, and will often thicken hair. Emu oil is an anti-inflammatory (topical and internal), very useful for pain relief and wound healing.

9. For stress reduction and improved sleep quality, **take supplements of a 10-amino acid ring from milk.**

10. For additional health benefits, **add concentrates made from multiple fruits and vegetables** (e.g., chlorophyll concentrates, flash-dried powdered fruit/vegetable supplements).

PART TWO

The MS Journey

This section is an invitation to those of you with MS in particular to take charge and impact your wellness. It goes deeper into the many practical physical, social, and psychological ramifications you encounter and can positively impact. Just a note, you will often hear Dr. Bill writing in the first person. That is because his personal perspective guides you through an experience and set of discoveries he knows intimately and firsthand.

PART TWO

The MS Journey

J ust a little background about MS. Multiple sclerosis, in its simplest
form, is believed to be an auto-immune disease. In short, some of
the body's own white blood cells are attacking the myelin (insulation
lining) of the nerve cells in the brain and spinal cord, or central nervous
system (CNS). Meanwhile, the nerves, muscle, and skin outside the CNS
are normal and are not under attack. Over time, the entire lining of the
myelin sheath may be removed and nerves are left without insulation.
This permits incorrect messaging to occur, or so-called "short-circuiting."
Eventually, many of these naked nerves or axons will die. This results in
impaired body movement and in some cases, paralysis.

Whenever injury occurs in our bodies, the body responds with an
attempt to heal itself using a process of inflammation, which includes
swelling, redness, heat, and pain or loss of function. This same process is
triggered whether it occurs in an ankle sprain or results from our own
white blood cells attacking tissue in the brain and spinal cord. The initial
problems with an attack of MS are usually partly or largely due to the
swelling component. This is why corticosteroids work, because, hopefully, they shorten the attack.

However, we also realize that corticosteroids do not benefit the illness of MS in the long term. This is an important distinction as it may
help the individual to decide whether or not to use corticosteroids. Of
course corticosteroids come with certain side effects such as early cataracts,
osteoporosis, peptic ulcers, mood changes, and even occasionally the

loss of a hip joint (avascular necrosis). The side effects are very important considerations in our cost-benefit decision, as in other parts of health and medicine.

When the body completes the inflammation process in its efforts to heal, we are left with the scar or sclerosis. A series of several scars in the CNS is described by the term *multiple sclerosis*. The scars show as white spots or patches on an image produced by magnetic resonance imaging (MRI).

How then can we as individuals control our MS? From the above description of the white blood cells attacking our nerves, inflammation, and eventual scarring, there are several steps where we may be able to influence things. Part Two addresses specific ways to:

1. Prevent what triggers the change in our white blood cell group.

2. Reduce the ability of this white blood cell group to gain access to the CNS (i.e., across the blood-brain barrier).

3. Reduce the inflammation and free radicals that damage the initial cells and also the surrounding cells.

4. Alter our diet to provide building blocks so injured cells in the CNS can be repaired or new healthy replacement cells can be generated.

Today, none of these can be accomplished completely or 100%. Hence, we must aim for partial improvement, with as few negative side effects as possible. If we can achieve several 10-15% pieces of the puzzle, then we can have an impact or start to control our illness. We are not talking about a cure. We are talking about making a difference to ourselves. Recognize that, over a period of 7-8 years, every single cell of our 70 trillion cells is replaced by a new cell.

It has recently been discovered that healing can occur in the brain and spinal cord; this has only been accepted in the last decade. One concession that multiple sclerosis does offer its victims is time. What we are suggesting is that it is up to the individual to empower him- or herself to make a difference in his or her own health. Thus, even if we are only

partly successful, we will still greatly enhance our outlook and, potentially, our outcome as well. The remainder of this section will outline
some of the steps that seem reasonable and have worked for others and
for me. None of the steps are harmful to anyone, and so there is little to
lose in trying them. The first principle learned in medical school is Hippocrates' statement, "Primum nom nocere"—"Do no harm." Every time
we use a drug in anesthesiology, it is with the concept of the risk-benefit ratio in mind. We follow that dictum in our everyday life, and this
book and the rest of Part Two aims to do this as well.

CHAPTER NINE

Dr. Bill's MS Journey

This chapter is dedicated to sharing more of my MS experiences. It covers how I arrived at this time of crisis in 1996 and how I emerged, making new dreams from shattered ones. It is in many ways illuminated by my earlier understanding of medicine and, naturally, because of my orientation, is slightly more technical in nature than other people's stories. Throughout Part Two you will hear me sporadically speaking intimately from my own voice when the storyline is personal and specific to my MS experiences.

Personal History

I am the fifth of seven children and was raised on a small, mixed farm in Saskatchewan. I left this small community to study medicine at the University of Saskatchewan in Saskatoon. Following this, I interned at St. Paul's Hospital in Saskatoon and completed an additional six months of anesthesia training. This was in preparation for a rural general practice with two colleagues in Hudson Bay, Saskatchewan. In my four years there, I diagnosed three people with multiple sclerosis and missed diagnosing at least one other.

In 1983, Denise and I decided to move to Calgary, where I would do a specialty in anesthesiology and intensive care. We moved with our two young sons, Warren and Brian, and in early 1984 were delighted at the birth of our daughter, Laura. During the five years in Calgary, I spent two years doing brain research. This involved lab work in the Department of Pharmacology and Anesthesiology as to how anesthetics worked on the brain, and it meant that my career was taking more of an academic turn. It was also at that time that I was fortunate enough to complete my board exams in both Canada and the United States.

Despite offers for further training at Stanford University in California and a clinical research position at MD Anderson Hospital in Houston, we decided to return to Saskatoon, where I joined the Faculty of Medicine. This started a delightful, and yet very hectic, four years. I became the Research Director in the Department of Anesthesiology and within a year had become the Residency Program Director as well. I continued to do research on the brain and was successful, along with several other colleagues, in attaining a $1 million research grant from the Heart and Stroke Foundation. However, at this same time, most of my health markers were deteriorating. My cholesterol continued to climb, my blood pressure was elevated, and my migraine headaches were so frequent I would use a large bottle of extra-strength acetaminophen every month.

In 1990, in Duncan, on Vancouver Island on the West Coast, I visited a colleague whom I had trained with in Calgary. He invited me to join him in clinical practice. In the spring of 1992, Denise and I decided to do just that. Prior to leaving Saskatoon, I was particularly impacted by the movie *Regarding Henry*, starring Harrison Ford. The message it conveyed to me was that, despite the huge problem Henry had with his health, his life actually improved when he stepped out of his hectic legal practice in New York. This was the first time I was able to admit to Denise that I was a workaholic.

A move at this time was a particular challenge for our older son, Warren, who was about to start high school. Even so, he was extremely generous and understanding. He said that we would make the right decision. I still appreciate his sensitivity and wisdom in accepting such a great change in our lives. By moving to the West Coast, I was, of course, leaving behind clinical research and clinical teaching. This meant my workload was decidedly less but permitted much more time to spend with my family. All of my stress-related health markers improved in that first year. In fact, the *Financial Post Fortune 500* magazine had a feature article on me, calling me the "Quintessential Baby Boomer." I was typical of the individual leaving his very hectic life in the city for a more relaxed laid-back life in a smaller center.

Like with many other addictions, a workaholic is only ever a "recovering workaholic," because we are never completely healed. This was certainly true for me. Within a year of moving to Vancouver Island, I started to see people for chronic and acute pain problems. This was almost always for one to three hours at the end of the day spent in the operating room.

Both chronic and acute pain issues are primarily concerned with the function of the nervous system. Two of my earliest patients had multiple sclerosis. One was helped with epidural injections that enabled her to sit down without extreme discomfort. The other had such severe muscle spasms that he had an infusion pump placed in his abdomen to deliver a drug, baclofen, continuously into his cerebrospinal fluid. At least once a month, I was responsible for refilling the pump with baclofen and supervising its delivery over 24 hours.

My ongoing interest in acute pain issues had resulted in my publishing a number of research articles and an editorial titled "Balanced Analgesia" in the *Canadian Journal of Anesthesiology*. My involvement with chronic pain, primarily while in private practice, resulted in my being invited to Australia in April 1996. I was one of the few Canadians asked to speak at the World Congress of Anesthesiology being held in Sydney. My topic was "How to Treat Pain Without the Use of Opiates" (narcotics). It was very exciting to be speaking to some 2,500 people, with pictures of myself across the front of the stage, leaving me nowhere to hide!

Changes and Symptoms

After returning home from the Congress of Anesthesiology, I started to notice that it was getting harder and harder to recover from my on-call nights. I was still cycling the six kilometers to work, but my right foot would frequently slip off the pedal and I would nearly fall. By early July, I chose to drive to and from work as a safer option. By then it was hard to recover from any day's work. I found it difficult to get up in the mornings and I remained groggy, despite going to bed at 9 or 10 o'clock at night. If it had been a busy call night in anesthesia and I was working most of a 24-hour period, even after an entire day of rest I did not feel recovered. In fact, I still didn't feel recovered by the time it was my turn to go back on-call again three days later.

I noticed other changes too. My right foot would slap at times when I walked, especially if I was tired. In addition, I was finding it more difficult to see my chronic pain clients for the usual two to three hours at the end of the operating room day. I had noticed a peculiar problem—the long, hollow needles I used for epidural injections seemed to be getting quite dull. I contacted the company's representative and she was very quick to send out two new boxes of needles. However, they were no better and it puzzled me.

Finally, in early July, I made an appointment for a checkup with my family doctor. She examined me and suggested I see a neurologist. I was seen soon thereafter by a University of British Columbia neurologist. He found many more signs and symptoms: significant hyperreflexia (over-reactive reflexes) on my right side, lateral gaze nystagmus, right-sided weakness, a positive Romberg's test, poor ability to track on the finger-to-nose test, and an inability to walk with one foot directly in front of the other. He also noted that I had a much-reduced sensation on my right side and that I was up three to four times a night to empty my bladder. By the end of the interview, he had booked me for an MRI. When he reviewed me two weeks later, he recommended I take six months off work because he believed I had multiple sclerosis.

I was devastated. So was my family. Denise and our older son, Warren, who were with me at the time of my Vancouver neurologist appointment, tried to support me. I said to Denise, "I feel like I am worth more dead than alive." I saw myself continuing to slide straight down the slope of diminished strength, balance, and energy. I anticipated progressive incapacity, even incontinence, needing to leave home for hospital, then an institution and early death. My neurologist believed that progressive multiple sclerosis was more probable, because my situation had worsened continuously over the last four months.

By the time I left work on August 23, 1996, I was having someone drive me to work. I stumbled around the operating room and seriously discussed with my coworkers the pros and cons of a three-wheel or four-wheel scooter for myself. I was unable to empty a syringe with my right hand, and both of my hands were so numb that procedures such as starting epidurals or intravenous needles were done solely on a visual basis. My diagnosis and major right-sided weakness explained one of my summer mysteries. I remembered that I had complained to the needle sales representative that their product seemed extraordinarily dull. The replacement needles had been no better. By the time I was diagnosed by the neurologist, the "penny had dropped." I realized that the epidural needles had been fine, but that the strength in my right hand had disappeared so gradually and insidiously that I had not realized that my hands were the problem.

COMMON SYMPTOMS OF MS

1. *Neuropathic pain*
2. *Cognitive "thinking" problems*
3. *Visual problems*
4. *Numbness and tingling*
5. *Bladder problems*
6. *Sexual changes*
7. *Loss of Balance*
8. *Fatigue*
9. *Muscle weakness, walking challenges*
10. *Muscle spasms*

For the next nine months, I continued to worsen. My depth of field vision (distance perception) was terrible. Even as a car passenger, I drove the driver to distraction and frustration. I worried that almost anyone would hit us at an intersection, or at a streetlight. I know now that 80% of multiple sclerosis patients are diagnosed with changes in their vision. Even though my case was not so severe, I now have a much better understanding of their fear and frustration.

Sleep: there was never enough. Even after 12-13 hours of rest, I would still feel like my arms and legs were nailed down to the bed. I often took an afternoon nap for one or two hours. One afternoon, as I awoke from my nap, I saw a hand in bed beside me. I had no concept of where this hand had come from. It was my hand. My whole sense of proprioception (aware-ness of where our limbs are) was almost gone. In fewer than six months, I'd gone from being able to play pretty fair ping-pong or tennis to having ter-rible eye-hand coordination.

Worse still, I was so irritable that after lunch my family would often specifically request that I have a nap. My uncontrollable irritability put tremendous stress on the relationships between my closest family members and myself. The chronic fatigue, coupled with my anger toward everything, especially myself, started to alienate my teenage sons, Brian and Warren. They became very reluctant to help me, no matter how small the request might be. My temper fuse was so short that they came to see my constant blowups as inevitable. My senses of vision, hearing, and even smell were so incredibly oversensitive that any small incident would trigger my anger. The term "naked nerve endings" was a common description and, in reality, I guess it was correct!

Family Challenges

I distinctly remember the 1996 Christmas season. Our immediate fam-ily decided to drive the 1,200 kilometers to Regina, Saskatchewan. This would enable Denise and me to see each of our siblings, and allow our kids to visit their cousins in both Regina and Calgary. To start, we took the ferry from Vancouver Island to Vancouver, British Columbia. It was dark by the time we docked at Tsawwassen terminal on the mainland side. Denise was driving and I was navigating (or at least trying to). We were supposed to meet and pick up our older son, Warren, who had just completed his first term at the University of British Columbia in Vancouver. Over the next 30 minutes, I proceeded to get Denise and our other two children hopelessly lost. Finally, our son Brian navigated. He was fed up with the recurrent bickering back and forth between Denise and me. I realized that there were more problems now than I had anticipated happening within my brain. My complete inability to navigate with the map both frustrated and frightened me; I had lost a significant skill, with which I had once excelled since my time as a Boy Scout. This was my first significant encounter with the cognitive component of multiple sclerosis.

Up to 60% of people with multiple sclerosis have significant cognitive problems. These include issues with problem solving, reading maps, short-term memory, and multitasking, as well as the development of what may be referred to as "brain fog."

With Brian at the wheel, we found Warren about 10 minutes later, but our trip did not improve. I was a major hassle and frustration to all my fellow travelers. I couldn't tolerate the flashing car lights, any kind of music jangled my ears, and I was soon very irritable, as even modest bumps in the road made sleep impossible for me. The bumps would trigger shooting electrical pain, with or without muscle spasms, into one or both legs. Seventy percent of people with multiple sclerosis suffer from one or both of these symptoms badly enough to seek medication or treatment. Unfortunately, this nerve irritability pain (neuropathic pain) is notoriously hard to treat. By the time we reached Regina, my family was almost ready to give me away. My multiple sclerosis had turned a happy trip into a near nightmare.

Facing Myself

When I returned to my neurologist in the New Year, it had been five months since my diagnosis and I was no better. In reality, I was worse than when I left work. My neurologist answered my question, "What do I do next?" with "You need to take another six months off." This statement made me realize two truths: 1) Western medicine has very little to offer chronic illness, and 2) if I were going to have any control over my recovery, then I would have to learn all I could about my illness.

I became aware of how fast and furious I had been running in my practice of medicine. It took months before I appreciated this little-known fact. Most of my medical colleagues routinely ran on a similar treadmill, resulting in great costs to themselves, their families, and eventually their own health. I've been told that the average lifespan of a physician in North America is 56 years; without a doubt, I know very few old anesthesiologists.

In February 1997, my dad was diagnosed with lymphoma, at the age of 79. At that time, I had already returned to my role as tenor in a local choir. My seatmate in the choir, a pathologist, remarked to me that my father's lymphoma was one of the nastiest and most aggressive cases he had ever seen. This was another major blow. My dad and I had always been extremely close. I decided not to discuss this grim prognosis with him. Instead, we six siblings (after losing a brother to AIDS in 1994) pulled together to support our parents. After many unsuccessful radiation treatments, my father gave chemotherapy a try. In addition to many hazardous side effects, this too proved ineffective. Several of us, including me, were starting to look outside traditional Western medicine in reaction to Dad's losing battle with cancer. However, we were unsuccessful. He passed away at home in mid-September of that year. For me it had seemed as though he had hung on until I had received back my hospital privileges, which came through two days before he died. This had been a goal of mine that had required several months of struggle to achieve, and he knew how important it was to me.

Following a week's refresher training in Victoria, I was booked for three successive Fridays to work in our local operating room, but by the third Friday I was much worse again. I had to recognize that something in the operating room milieu was having a negative impact on my health. Had I proved myself wrong regarding anesthesia and its "non-worsening" of MS symptoms? Absolutely. This was another bitter pill to swallow. Maybe, just maybe, I had to look beyond the regular boundaries of accepted medical practice for relief of my own progressive multiple sclerosis.

By now it was the latter part of 1997. I had learned of an upcoming conference in Vancouver about complementary and alternative methods to either slow down MS symptoms or assist my tolerance of them. I attended, and the conference was a whole new experience. I was placed with a large number of people who had multiple sclerosis, at all stages and ages. I felt very lucky to still be able to walk, albeit with a limp. More importantly, I realized that many others were seeking new options in their own journey with this chronic illness.

New Options and Possibilities

The conference proved to be my introduction to the Paleolithic Diet or Stone Age Diet, which I then went on. I stayed on it for almost a month and then, not seeing any changes, I gave it up. However, it did make a huge impact on me insofar as convincing me of the possibility that I might be able to control my MS. Denise and I started to look at diet changes we could implement or what particular nutritional supplements might make a difference in my multiple sclerosis.

Certainly, the first change or improvement on my road to recovery was reduced fatigue. Admittedly, this was a small baby step, but I became better at seeing and appreciating small changes. Not being quite as exhausted was the first improvement, which I attributed to the teaspoon of emu oil I was taking in the hope that its anti-inflammatory effect would benefit me. Coupled with this was slightly longer ability to stand, before needing to sit down. However, I still dragged my right leg and could "trip" without reason.

Somewhere, about April 1997, most of my light touch returned. I attributed this to intravenous chelation by my naturopath, after he determined from a urine and hair sample that I had an excess of lead, a heavy metal. My clarity of thinking also improved. However, it took five more months for me to regain my hospital privileges.

The regaining of my hospital privilege required legal assistance and was coupled with my dad's cancer and, in September 1997, his death. My anesthesia colleagues even required a psychiatric statement of my well-being and adequacy of mental health. This was particularly devastating to Denise in that all my depression and personal health issues had quickly traversed our small community. Yes, I was angry, too, perhaps more so with myself, for my sharing the personal matter of my depression with friends and colleagues. However, I was nearly numb with frustration and primarily wanted to be able to restart my anesthesia career or "life." Finally, push came to shove, somewhere, and I started back to work on a temporary basis in late 1997.

My hand numbness returned after three successive Fridays back in the operating room. My family doctor advised against further anesthesia practice and I realized she was right, albeit, not permanently, just then. The hospital administration and my anesthesiology "friends and colleagues" nailed down the coffin some four weeks later. This was achieved with some careful and complicit manipulation of dates and paperwork on their part. This confirmed my decision to discontinue working, as I would have to start at the beginning as a new applicant for anesthesiology staff privileges—full time or nothing. I knew I was beat, so I quit banging my head against the wall.

Crisis

My next option was a civil suit against my anesthesiology colleagues and the hospital. Unfortunately, this would have had to be completely on my own nickel. The Canadian Medical Protective Association would have had to defend the practicing anesthesiology individual in this scenario. Sure, Denise and I were really angry and hurt. My family and I wanted fairness, restitution, and even revenge. But, we were financially broke as well, and a long, slow legal process would be very expensive. In addition, I might only achieve another chance to resume my anesthesiology practice. My health may not have permitted success with another try. I finally said,

"Enough!" and moved on from needing to resume my medical career to the recognition that my health and my family were more important. This painful step was a critical turning point in my personal health journey. I hope that my sharing it here will help you to make the correct decisions for yourself. Would I do it differently now, seven years later? Possibly. Could or can I? Probably not.

Personal crisis, whether physical, mental, or emotional, can contribute to our health journey. Often letting go of our anger and/or allowing forgiveness can resolve the crisis. The only person we can truly control is ourselves. Those around us are factors we can possibly influence a little, but never control.

Despite this insight, the touch in my hands has never returned. In fact, I have lost light touch on my entire body. Maybe, just maybe, it has improved on my left side in the past few months. I believe this is possible because several of my health choices will continue to reduce the toxins within me. These include lots of purified water, glutathione building blocks, organic and/or natural foods, and an organic-origin multivitamin/multi-mineral. Coupled with these are exposure to clean air, water, and environment, as much as possible.

Hope and Improvement

Small steps of improvement occurred over the next four years. Emu oil, plenty of ground flax, rest, reduced stress, and the life cycle on our small acreage were part of this gradual blunting of my super-sensitivity to sound, motion, and smell. I regained my balance. My migraine headaches became much less frequent when I gave up wheat that contained the subset of gluten called gliadin. I suspect this may have reduced one of my MS triggers. To the personal list of foods to avoid, I have added cheese, milk, yogurt, wine with sulfites (as preservatives), and scotch whiskey. I will occasionally cheat and have ice cream. Also, I still take four pouches of whey protein isolate daily. It has no casein or fatty acids in it, and therefore does not have the possible MS trigger in it called butyrophilin. This should reassure most of us who are in agreement with the important items to avoid in our diet relative to the Paleolithic Diet.

The next major piece of the puzzle was my learning about this whey protein isolate as a useful building block for glutathione in every cell. As of late 2001, I started on a packet or envelope every day for three months. I noticed no difference. However, after speaking to research scientists in eastern Canada, I increased this to three packets per day. Their premise was that by the time a person is diagnosed with a major neurodegenerative disease such as MS or Parkinson's, the glutathione in his or her body cells could be as low as 5% of normal.

Happily, within a month of being on three packages a day, my energy began to significantly improve. Within another two to three months, I had enough energy to book in with a personal trainer to recover some of my strength, balance, and coordination. Over four months I made steady progress, to both my surprise and everyone else's. My right leg limp almost disappeared. My muscle strength improved, and my need to sit down soon after standing almost disappeared. I could walk considerable distances! You can imagine my sense of well-being five years after losing most of these abilities. I wanted to talk about hope again with MS, rather than just endure the inevitable.

My pain and muscle spasms started to recede, until after six months on three packets a day they were nearly gone. I had some slight improvement in mental clarity and cognitive ability, but only minimal. However, my hypersensitivity to smells, sounds, and "bumps" on the road while in a car diminished a fair bit. My disappointment in my lack of cognitive ability was tempered somewhat, as I had already learned that cognitive impairment is only slightly linked to the degree of physical disability. My sense of touch has not improved, but I can live with that.

By late 2002, I had found a short-term energy tonic that worked to enhance focus and concentration for several hours. By now, I had given up coffee, tea, and cola drinks because they left me feeling jangled and shaky, plus they gave me diarrhea. Caffeinated products often cause flare-ups in those with irritable bowel syndrome. This herbal energy tonic acutely raises potassium and magnesium. It also contains guarana, a slow 6- to 8-hour burn xanthine. As noted, it has similar effects to caffeine, but causes fewer high spikes and is more sustained.

Now I am up to the toilet to void or empty my bladder once or twice a night. I have had half as many trips at night while on a high-quality saw palmetto product, also containing damiana, ginseng, and ginkgo biloba. It is now understood that saw palmetto calms many of our irritable bladder receptors. Hence, it is equally indicated in both men and women with MS. I still need to double void (i.e., make two trips) to empty my bladder more completely. (If bladder infections, especially in women, are commonplace, refer to Chapter 14: Sexuality and Bladder Issues.)

The general heat sensitivity of our brain and spinal cord tissues is the reason so many of us with MS avoid sunlight. As mentioned previously, avoiding bright sunlight costs us vitamin D and optimal melatonin production. This awareness of injured brain vulnerability is also of concern in regards to the use of general anesthesia drugs. I suggest MS people consider spinal, epidural, or regional anesthesia (freezing the nerves) whenever possible. In recent years anesthesiologists have also leaned in this direction. If fear of "being awake" is your issue, they have many other choices to temporarily transport you to "never, never land." Please recall my two years in lab research on how general anesthetics has influenced my approach to this general anesthesia (GA) issue. Personal stories I have heard include a gerontologist asking six elderly Nobel Prize winners how long after a GA before they felt their brain worked normally again. They averaged six months in their replies. I believe caution in any brain illness or injury is prudent.

Issues involving my cognitive problems bear further comment as well. First, I continue to improve, even if only slightly, a little at a time, month by month. I do not know if this is brain recovery or improved adaptation or even recruitment of other parts of the brain. It may even be a composite of all three. I do know my creativity is slightly better, as is my patience. These compensate somewhat for the concrete linear clarity of problem solving I once enjoyed.

Getting Feedback

Of interest, in 2002 I was asked by my disability insurance company to have an independent assessment done by an expert in MS at Scripps Clinic, La Jolla, California. My medical records, including my MRI preceded me. This very experienced neurologist was quite impressed with my degree of recovery. In noting this to me, he asked what I felt my toughest problem was. I replied, "Brain fog." He was having none of this and wanted a detailed explanation. I did my best to explain my lack of multi-tasking, my poor quality short-term memory, and so on. He was not enamored with my ability to put this in scientific terms. Then he sent me for his pet or "favourite" test on cognitive function. This was a timed performance of addition and subtraction of the second or third last number. I did fair at the gentle speed, abysmally at the normal speed, and even worse at a moderately faster speed. He seemed completely able to accept my explanation once he saw the objective data.

Now, many of you would say, aren't they going to give me a similar second chance, for a second opinion? My own neurologist, Dr. Don Paty, here in Canada, had already told me it was quite unusual to fly someone to an expert in another country. Dr. Paty was one of a handful of experts on MS on the planet. You could also ask, was I at my best? Well, no, I do not want to be "at my best" but more typically should be at my worst when being assessed. Neither you nor I have any control of our best and worst days. Hence, when assessed or completing paperwork we need to record our worst-case scenarios. Why? Because almost every disability is seen as static or fixed. Woe to you if you take the Pollyanna or "best possible day" approach. Certainly, denial is your option, but if your healthcare practitioner and disability assessor are going to be able to fairly assess you, this is the only recommendation I can give you.

An interesting parallel to this is your own history of previous MS attacks recalled from your memory. These attacks mean much less than those episodes documented by a physician at the time. Please remember that. This advice may help you a great deal in the challenging financial journey you are on with this multiple sclerosis (or other chronic illness) diagnosis. My experienced family physician tried to end on an optimistic note as to my potential recovery. The agencies reviewing your case will always hook on to this "reduced disability" and go there, *not* to where you are.

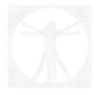

CHAPTER TEN

Dr. Bill's Healthy Discoveries/Food Sensitivities

As discussed, in November 1997 I attended the MS Society of Canada's Conference in Vancouver for Complementary and Alternative Choices for MS. This proved to be an important key to my modest recovery from MS. One of my sisters in Calgary had seen an ad discussing the conference and had alerted me. I had not heard anything about the conference despite living on Vancouver Island, only two hours from Vancouver. Of course, neither had I joined a local MS support group then. At this stage I believe I was using denial and withdrawing from others as a means of coping.

My family doctor, always very thorough and supportive, had probably told me about the local support group—but it went by me. In reality, most items went "by me," due to my loss of concentration and focus from MS. Approximately 60-70% of folks with MS have varying degrees of cognitive or "thinking" problems. At this time, I was not even reading the local newspaper, which announced the monthly MS support group meetings in my town. Actually, it was in registering for this Vancouver conference with MS Canada's British Columbia provincial office that my contact with the local MS Society was initiated.

I phoned the toll-free number in Vancouver and explained that I wanted to attend the MS conference. The woman in the office asked if I was a member of an MS Society. "No," I said, and asked what difference that would make. She explained it was $100 for physicians, but only $10 for members. Well, money was still very scarce for us at this time so I asked if I could join now and still qualify for the $10 conference fee. She agreed and wrote down my name, address, and phone number so that an employee of the MS Society of Vancouver Island could follow up. Indeed, it was meeting this Occupational Therapist for coffee three to four weeks later that started me on another key part of my journey.

At the Vancouver conference, I looked around the room on Saturday morning and was surprised at the wide spectrum of people nearly filling the room. Many looked normal, while others looked challenged with a degree of disability. In reality, some of the "normal looking" had MS and others were family members or healthcare practitioners (nurses, social workers, physiotherapists, occupational therapists, even an occasional MD) interested in MS.

The majority of attendees were young women, not surprising when 70% of people with MS are women and many of the interested healthcare practitioners are also women. Space and bathrooms were at a premium. About half of the folks in wheelchairs were men. By now I had learned that even though fewer men had MS, more of them are severely affected and their MS is often more rapidly progressive.

The presentations were varied, from medical descriptions of MS to unique and particular therapies in smaller groups. Several people presented testimonials of their individual successes. I believe that these were especially useful to many of us with MS. Why? Because they were from the heart and expressed "hope" to the audience: Maybe I can recover some as well!

The symptom management sessions were helpful. One session presented healing and "retraining" or "recruiting" motor nerve pathways according to work by Meir Schneider. Another session, the most memorable for me, discussed the use of the Chinese medicine moxibustion for pain and fatigue management.

However, the session that had the most impact on me long term was related to the potential dietary triggers of multiple sclerosis and a discussion of the Stone Age or Paleolithic Diet—the diet people had prior to 15,000-

20,000 years ago. This was presented by Matt Embry, a twenty-year-old man from Calgary with multiple sclerosis. I also met his parents, who were with him. His mother had a degree in nursing and worked in public health. His father, Ashton Embry, who had a PhD in geology and worked for the National Research Council, had done an exhaustive study of all the existing MS literature. His son had been diagnosed with severe MS at the age of 18.

From his family's research, Matt explained that diet was thought to play a key role in triggering and probably aggravating MS. He explained that grains and dairy products were often triggers of MS, through a process of "molecular mimicry"; that is, a portion of the protein in the grain or dairy product was similar to that of the myelin surrounding the nerves. This protein portion escapes from the gastrointestinal tract and enters the blood stream. Because this protein is viewed by the body as being foreign, the body mounts a defense against the protein. Because the protein also looks like (mimics) the myelin protein, the body also attacks the myelin. Because of this error by the body, Matt explained, his family followed a reasonably restrictive diet with rice as the only grain, bananas, fish, white meat (chicken breast), and a few other foods. Based on the information presented by Matt and from my discussion with his parents, I decided to look at the Stone Age or Paleolithic Diet.

Our current modern diet is a far cry from the Paleolithic Diet. At that time (prior to 10,000 years ago), humans ate 200 different "whole foods" per year. This included a very wide variety of fruits and vegetables, game meat, and fish. Game meat and fish were sources of high-quality protein and provided small amounts of saturated fat. It was extremely rare for people to have excess or even abundant fat, except for coastal fishing people. Grains were limited to small grass seeds, as this was prior to the Agricultural Revolution and grains had not yet become a large part of our diet.

Diet Insights

Paleolithic people had a large intake of green vegetables and plants. This resulted in a large amount of omega-3 fatty acids being consumed. It is believed that we used to eat a much higher ratio of omega-3 to omega-6 fats, 1:1 or 1:2. But today, as Chapter 7 outlines, many of us are 1:18 or 1:20 in our intake of omega-3s to omega-6s because of our high oil intake of corn, safflower, and soybean oil, and other oil crops.

Also as noted in Chapter 7, because omega-3 oils easily go rancid, they are not usually used in commercially produced foods. Consequently, omega-6 oils, which are hydrogenated or modified, are used in baked goods, most margarines, and almost all fried foods. These modified oils have a longer shelf life and do not taste rancid. However, they also contain harmful trans fats. And, as we now know, trans fats are extremely harmful to our health and should be avoided!

Dr. Peter J. d'Adamo's book *Eat Right 4 Your Blood Type* is a good place to start for understanding our need for dietary individualization. Certainly, determining blood type is one of the first steps when deciding upon organ transplants. A very good friend of mine who has 12 years of education in Food Science is truly converted to the validity of food selection according to blood type. We should at least examine where we fit in. I am blood type A, which is suggested to be primarily vegetarian. Yet, I personally do better without wheat. That is a paradoxical statement for a Western Canadian prairie farm boy! Fortunately, Dr. d'Adamo's book provides sufficient detail for foods to be minimized in the diets of people such as myself with type A blood.

Other means to determine food sensitivities include VEGA testing and the ELISA blood test. In my first book, *Youth Renewed: A Common Sense Approach to Vibrant Health...at Any Age*, I discuss the VEGA machine with modest enthusiasm. I now believe it is only a guide and can lead to misinterpretation. Similarly, the ELISA blood test is not perfect either. This blood collection tests for antibodies to particular foods, and in my discussions with many naturopaths I have heard that the testing labs are considerably hampered by available consistency of the base foods. In addition, occasional contaminants such as dust, herbicides, and pesticides, or even peanuts, a common antigen, can skew the results incorrectly.

I admit I am weak with strict diets. I lasted only five weeks on the Embry's version of the Paleolithic Diet. Next, Denise and I set up a progressive elimination diet for me at home. I carefully spent two weeks on it but learned nothing. I found this discouraging, as the "elimination diet" is considered the gold standard for "food sensitivity" by clinical and allergy research dieticians. In retrospect, I should have continued on the elimination diet for at least four more weeks.

Food Sensitivities Reveal Themselves

Then, I got lucky and discovered the primary trigger of my frequent migraines. By then, our son Warren was attending the University of British Columbia. Like many college students, he had found the cheapest acceptable beer with the highest percentage of alcohol of 7%, produced by a small brewery in Saskatoon. Needless to say, I was delighted when Warren brought some of this beer home one weekend. Finally, the shoe of who purchased the beer was partly on the other foot!

However, much to my chagrin, whenever I drank one of the 7% beers, I would get a migraine headache. Ironically, I could drink two 5% beers without getting a headache. The difference? Wheat. The extra sugars or carbohydrates in a beer made with wheat permit a higher alcohol content. Eureka! I gave up wheat thereafter. This included all modern wheat such as that in bread, buns, pasta, breakfast cereals, and many processed foods. Denise taught me how to read food labels in order to eliminate wheat, wheat flour, wheat gluten, durum, and even semolina from my diet. Wheat is by far the most common grain in Canada and the northern United States. It is therefore an important component of many foods or snacks—including many chocolate bars!

I soon found that if I cheated or made an error reading labels, I paid for it with a major migraine. This encouraged me to carefully select foods. As a bonus, I soon lost 10 pounds (4.5 kg) of weight! Many, many foods in North America contain some sort of wheat component.

I learned about spelt, an old wheat farmed until the late 1950s in Saskatchewan and now back in demand, especially in British Columbia.

Kamut is also an old wheat (theoretically from King Tutankhamun's tomb of ancient Egypt, opened in the 1900s). Many of our friends on Canada's west coast, especially women, avoid wheat. They have found they feel better without it in their diet.

Similarly, when visiting health food stores in Kitchener, Waterloo (just southwest of Toronto), I learned more supportive data. One store-owner told me that many Germans and Austrians had immigrated to this region of Canada. However, most of them found they could not tolerate Canada's wheat bread or pasta. Consequently, there is a thriving spelt and kamut bakery and pasta niche in Kitchener-Waterloo. This trend toward the use of spelt flour is seen in other Canadian cities, including Vancouver, Victoria, and Toronto.

THREE MAJOR FOOD SENSITIVITIES IN THE WESTERN DIET

1. *Wheat*

2. *Milk*

3. *Red kidney beans*

The lectins in these foods result in the body's sensitivity to them.

The short story is, whichever grain is dominant in a society, a number of people will be "sensitized" to it. Hence, the major grain sensitivity in Mexico is corn, and in Asia, rice.

At the second British Columbia MS Society Complementary Medicine Conference in Vancouver in 2002, Denise and I learned more about why wheat and other foods were linked with MS. Our favourite speaker at that second conference was Dr. Lynn Toohey, of Colorado, United States. She has her PhD and has specialized in research of the Paleolithic Diet. She explained about lectins, a small but important component that can trigger auto-immune diseases, particularly MS. Lectins are found in many foods including grains (e.g., wheat, barley), legumes (e.g., kidney beans, soybeans, peanuts), plants of the nightshade family (e.g., potatoes, tomatoes, peppers), and dairy. Lectins contain both protein and sugar. They are able to bind to the outside of a cell, including the lining of the gut, and cause biochemical changes in it. Thus, they can interfere with digestion and absorption in our gut. They can also damage the gut lining. Therefore, food proteins and lectins can then enter our bloodstream. These can then trigger auto-immune diseases.

In light of this, I reduced my milk product intake, which seemed to further reduce my migraine headaches. I already knew I was lactose intolerant, so I had eliminated dairy products on an empty stomach unless I had lactase enzymes with me. I admit, I still cheat occasionally and eat ice cream and milk chocolate. I have never noted an issue with red kidney beans or soy products, but have minimized these, too. A further key point on diet that I have recently had confirmed is the importance of digestive enzymes. Previously, I thought I only needed Lactaid with lactase, or Beano with some carbohydrate digestive enzymes. One or both of these would usually reduce my gastric hurry, diarrhea, abdominal cramps, and excess rectal gas (flatus). I now know that a quality, general digestive enzyme containing amylase, protease, lipase, and lactase is beneficial for me and many other people, especially as we age.

Earlier Denise had taught me that fat is a common trigger of heartburn rather than extra stomach acidity. I agree, as a digestive enzyme before or with fatty foods protects me from heartburn. It is now accepted that acid reflux into the lower esophagus is usually due to a relative relaxation or opening of the lower esophagus sphincter ("valve"). Nearly all fat seems to loosen this physiologic valve with consequent heartburn. Hence, if the digestive enzyme lipase is used, heartburn is often avoided.

Enzymes for Digestion

The further advantage of taking plant digestive enzymes with almost every meal is that this helps to compensate for the gradual reduction in acid secretion in the stomach that occurs as we get older. The decrease in stomach acid begins at about age 40 and continues as we age. Taking digestive enzymes is very important for optimizing our food digestion with enzymes secreted by the pancreas and gallbladder. Otherwise, we will not get the maximum benefit from our food and may experience further unpleasant side effects, such as diarrhea, rushing for a bowel movement, abdominal cramps, and strong, often foul-smelling gas per rectum (flatus).

A couple, originally from England, were delighted with this knowledge we shared with them. He had started to describe himself as the "Fart King of Vancouver Island." She had given up her favorite food, fish and chips, as she got either heartburn or abdominal pain whenever she ate them. Once they took two digestive enzymes prior to or with their meals, both troubles almost completely resolved. She can eat fish and chips as much as she wishes now!

I recently learned about another benefit of digestive enzymes when I was in southern Ontario. A friend had booked me for an appointment with a well-trained and experienced live blood cell microscopist, whose background included over 20 years of clinical and research lab experience in a hospital. The day I visited this microscopist, my breakfast, two hours earlier, had been a cheese and vegetable omelet and toast, with no enzymes. I was appalled at the incredible clumping (major and excess rouleaux formation) of my red blood cells. She then had me take three large capsules, removing the coating to speed the benefit, with 10 ounces of reverse osmosis water. She took another fresh sample of blood 25 minutes later. The microscope revealed an incredible improvement. I now had little or no clumping of my red blood cells! Recurrent clumping and reduced blood flow can definitely worsen your chances of a heart attack or stroke.

After this experience, I was deeply convinced about the benefits of digestive enzymes and will always add them to my regimen. If you are over 40, or have MS, I would recommend a similar pattern. Europeans, especially Germans, have expounded on the value of these digestive enzymes. Wise use of such enzymes will likely pay for itself by further nutritive value absorbed from the food we eat. In addition, many unpleasant gut troubles may well be minimized, possibly even "leaky gut syndrome."

What is leaky gut syndrome and why should we care? This very common health disorder is thought to be due to local injury to the cells that line the small intestine. Keep in mind that our small bowel is 20-30 feet in length. This injury to the cells causes them to swell. Consequently, this reduces the "tight" contact between cells and allows undigested food particles to leak into the blood circulation.

Many things can cause this type of injury. Major irritants are believed to be "food sensitive" or "allergic proteins" such as wheat or cow's milk proteins. Repeated insult from eating these proteins will worsen the gut "leakiness." Foods containing lectins can also damage the small intestine, leading to a leaky gut. Small pieces of proteins and lectins can now directly enter the bloodstream. Several consequences result from this ongoing, foreign protein "leak" through the gut lining and into the blood. First, a set of white blood cells and their particular cell line is sensitized to the protein and increasingly expanded in numbers. Then, some secondary trigger, most likely viral but possibly some other toxin (e.g., herbicide or pesticide), foreign protein, vaccination, or something else of dietary origin causes a change in the white blood cells. Now this entire cell line of white blood cells is "permanently confused" and responds to a "similar looking" but *different body protein*. If this protein is the lining of joints or synovium, we get rheumatoid arthritis. If the protein looks like the protein lining of our myelin in our brain and spinal cord, we get multiple sclerosis. The term for some of our white cells attacking one of our tissues is *molecular mimicry*.

One common group of drugs, the NSAID (non-steroidal anti-inflammatory drugs)—such as ibuprofen, ASA, naproxen, and diclofenac—definitely can cause, or worsen, leaky gut syndrome. This is partly why they trigger gut bleeding in many of us. Local infections in the gut (bacteria from food poisoning or viral infections) can also cause a leaky gut.

Close cousins of the NSAIDs are the COX-2 inhibitors, such as Vioxx and Celebrex. They, too, may have similar side effects. As a result, I avoid taking these medications and reach for acetaminophen (paracetomol in some countries), opiates (narcotics), or other painkillers. In addition, these same NSAIDs and COX-2 inhibitors are now considered responsible for slow healing in our bodies. Virtually all healing of skin, brain, joints, and gut have an inflammatory component to healing that is hindered and/or slowed down by this group of drugs. Sadly, repeated use of these drugs or the cortisone group shortens our time before needing joint replacement or other surgical solutions, by reducing our body's ability to heal.

The other necessary component in multiple sclerosis is the "leaky blood-brain barrier" associated with MS. Perhaps this foreign protein in the bloodstream reacts against these Blood Brain Barrier (BBB) cells similar to the gut lining. Now they have "holes" and it is through these that this sensitized white blood cell line passes to be able to attack the myelin lining of the nerves in the brain and spinal cord. As alluded to earlier, wheat protein and milk protein are the two most likely triggers of MS that act in this fashion.

In reviewing the incidence of MS and geographical distribution, especially across the northern United States and Canada, questions come to mind. With the incidence of MS being greater in some areas, and not others, we need some additional explanation for these differences other than just vitamin D and less sun exposure. I suggest that the high preponderance in the Midwest or prairies is the incredible intake of modern wheat and wheat pasta in the "bread basket" region. In the recent MS Canada study, the other region highest in MS is the Maritimes or Atlantic region. I would have expected this region to get some protection from a reasonably high fish oil and omega-3 intake. However, I suspect the very high preponderance of polluted air, water, and soil may be the contributing factor. The prevailing winds from the Great Lakes industrial region and polluted air from the eastern seaboard of the United States may combine to worsen MS incidence in Atlantic Canada. In short, food sensitivities play a role in MS, but so does the quality of our air, water, soil, food, and environment.

In summary, food sensitivities and dietary components can trigger MS and other illnesses. Thus, current research supports eliminating wheat, cow's milk, and lectins from the diet. I, too, recommend these dietary changes, but I do differ with respect to cow's milk. I believe dietary casein—the protein used in making cheese—should be eliminated. However, I also believe that a particular pharmaceutical or specialized whey protein isolate from cow's milk is beneficial. In my review of data, my understanding is that a milk protein bound to milk fat (butyrophilin) may be a trigger of "molecular mimicry." The connection between butyrophilin and MS has been reported in the scientific literature. Because this specialized whey protein is fat-free, the risk of butyrophilin being present to trigger MS is remote. Furthermore, many people with MS have had considerable improvement in their symptoms from taking this specialized whey protein. This has also been noted by Dr. Lynn Toohey, who specializes in dietary triggers of today's auto-immune illnesses.

If you have MS or other chronic illness, I would encourage you to consider food sensitivities as being part of the problem. Try an elimination diet to determine which foods may be giving you problems. Eliminating certain foods from your diet can be challenging, but it just might help. Check with your Department of Health or medical center to find a qualified dietician or nutritionist to help you with your elimination diet. You need to know which foods you can eat and which supplements to take so that your dietary intake is healthy and balanced in nutrients.

CHAPTER ELEVEN

The MS Society, Networks, and Wellness

All of us tend to underestimate the importance of our interaction with other human beings. Indeed, having an illness such as MS often diminishes relationships within your workplace and even in your community. For me, my busy medical practice, including operating room anesthesiology, acute pain rounds, and chronic pain outpatients, dramatically reduced my interpersonal contacts outside of work. This was obvious and necessary due to the tremendous fatigue I was experiencing due to the MS. My MS also put a strain on my interaction with medical colleagues, as they no longer knew how to interact with me.

It took me awhile to admit how much I, too, need relationships and personal interaction to operate fully as a human being. Maybe part of this need comes from being the fifth of seven children. Perhaps it developed through my enjoyment of 65 classmates in medical school and 15-20 colleagues during internship and anesthesia residency. This social gap caused by MS was gradually filled by my involvement with the local MS Society support group, my MS Society Board participation, and even national and some international participation.

Much of my new social involvement began as a result of the effort and energy expended on me by Helen Catherall, an occupational therapist employed part-time by the Vancouver Island MS Society. She met me at a local restaurant for coffee and spent time building my sense of well-being. She started with simple physical and emotional issues. She suggested our family meet with the MS chapter social worker to establish a baseline of how each of us was coping with my MS diagnosis and changes. She also addressed my difficulties with the disability pension plan application and refusals. She diplomatically outlined why an automobile handicapped parking sign or sticker could save my meager energy supply. Finally, she described the function of the local MS Society and Board and how I could be helpful to them. The latter was partly due to my research and grantsmanship experience in brain and stroke research on two university campuses. This helped my self-esteem by demonstrating to me that I could still be of value to my community.

Becoming a Team Player

Soon after being introduced to Helen, I began to come out of my self-imposed isolation and withdrawal—I began to move on from "poor me" or "no-value me" to becoming a team player again in the game of life. For example, the handicap parking sticker was useful, both for parking and for me recognizing that I was part of a "challenged" or "special needs" group. It was also a part of my "coming out" or admitting to others that I had a chronic illness. This is a tough step for many of us. I have met people who have "closeted" their MS for 5-20 years. Certainly denial is a useful defense mechanism, but even more important is the next step of personal interaction, cooperative education, support, and, yes, the power of new friendships.

I still remember the relief of parking near the door of the grocery store. Yes, I could have a little extra energy to push the grocery cart! I had already learned that a grocery cart was an "invisible" walking aid, acceptable to others and myself. My daughter, Laura, was initially hesitant to ride with me and park in a handicap-parking stall. She either did not see me as handicapped or did not want to accept me as such. In time, this hesitance eased. I learned that even big changes start with small steps, literally.

Soon after meeting Helen, I went to my first local MS support group. This was pretty traumatic. Two-thirds of the regular group were using canes, walkers, or wheelchairs. I also saw a man I had sung tenor with in choir for three years. He, too, had just been diagnosed with MS. One of the more outspoken members of the group approached me boldly and insisted I should sign up to work at the local bingo hall to help support the group through gaming. She stated I should get at it right away, as I was still walking. I have always been poor at saying no and this was no exception. Thankfully, my mom later offered to fill this time slot in the smoke-filled bingo hall. I sometimes forget the great support I have received. Unfortunately, meeting a high proportion of people who were walking-challenged further skewed my long-term outlook and hope. To this point, I mostly had seen MS-compromised individuals in a hospital setting, and seeing them in a community setting did nothing to raise my spirits.

Join a Group

Helen's visit also led to my introduction to Paul McNamara, the Executive Director of the Victoria-based MS Society Chapter. He was fairly new in his role there and was looking for Society Board members to fill particular needs. We hit it off well and he introduced me to a large set of useful and supportive resources. Helen and Paul soon had me enrolled in a 12-member, newly diagnosed group. This was led by Bonnie Pashak, a talented and passionate social worker of the MS Society. Within two months, I was a new Board member representing my area of Duncan and fulfilling the role of novelty specialist physician with a neuroscience research background and his own MS.

Our newly diagnosed group, led by Bonnie, gelled quickly into friendships, trust, and mutual support. We were all hungry for stories similar to our own so that we could realize we were "not the only one" with this peculiar fate. The group was two-thirds women and one-third men—representative of the population of MS in Canada. We shared the "but you look so well" that we had all heard so frequently, and we laughed at it. We often cried over other issues of emotional pain and work trials and tribulations. I suspect that it was this emotional roller coaster, which Bonnie guided so patiently, that bonded us together so quickly. In fact, we continued to meet for nearly two years, and some of us are still close friends seven years later. Only now do I fully appreciate the significance of these contacts. Interaction of like-minded or similarly challenged people makes for more powerful individuals and a unique team approach. Yes, laughter is still the best medicine. I believe most of us started our recovery and our renewed belief in ourselves in this group. Certainly, I did. This group, the newly diagnosed or newly accepting of a diagnosis of MS, also helped our primary and secondary caregivers in a positive fashion.

Check Out the MS Society

A concurrent event in my journey was becoming a Board member in the MS Society chapter based in Victoria. My interaction with this group also became a valuable experience in my journey toward wellness. The Board represented some 1,300 folks with MS, of a total population of 700,000 people on Vancouver Island. It is one of the most physically and emotionally supportive and rehabilitative options in North America. This got my attention, big time. After sliding downhill steadily for 13 months, I felt I needed an option for family respite, in case the rapid slide continued. Victoria had a 100-110 MS client caseload of frequent and regular visits to the MS centre. The benefits derived were dramatic and enabled many to stay in their own home and out of institutional care. I admit I wanted to become a part of this group rather than run the risk of burdening my family with my total care or face the possibility of being institutionalized.

In late 1997 my long-term prognosis looked dismal. The rapid advance of my progressive multiple sclerosis was unrelenting. I have a habit of wanting to have all my bases covered. I felt that as an active member, I had a good chance of slipping into this long-established core group. Each year, one or two of our members with MS would need to retire from the group due to the worsening of their MS. I did not know when my own number would come up. I had no idea, or long-term hope, of being as recovered as I am today!

More Personal Challenges

As a chapter member in the autumn of 1998, I was asked to attend the International Symposium of Multiple Sclerosis in Cleveland, Ohio. I was excited at the prospect, believing I would discover the latest and greatest options for treatment and rehabilitation of MS. Three weeks prior to this I tried riding a recumbent bicycle previously ridden across Canada by Pierre Doré. After only 10 feet, I stopped, fell over, and badly smashed my right ankle. This occurred in a back alley in downtown Vancouver. My friends helped me into a van and drove me to nearby St. Paul's Hospital. However, I should have tied my feet together with my shoelaces, as I had learned in Boy Scout First Aid. Once placed on the floor of the van, my right foot plunked over at a right angle to my body, because no bony or tissue support remained! I was fortunate to see a "Top Gun" orthopedic surgeon, Dr. Simon Horlick, who explained I needed two pieces of steel and five to six months of non-weight-bearing time (i.e., a wheelchair). Membership in the medical profession does have its privileges; Dr. Horlick asked me if I had any requests in my 28-36 hours' wait for an emergency surgery slot. I asked to see an anesthesiologist from the Acute Pain service. My "wish" was granted and he set me up with a push button pump for morphine (PCA or Patient Controlled Analgesic) and a twice-daily dose of oral naproxen, 500 mg. The two in combination are quite good for bone and soft tissue injury pain control. Just when I thought I was on cloud nine (morphine has been nicknamed "nectar of the gods") I had a rude awakening. The combination of being bedridden, on a tricyclic antidepressant, and now morphine, plus my MS meant I could not empty my bladder. This necessitated urinary catheterization by a young, embarrassed nurse. I had the catheter for several days, almost right up until the time I was discharged from hospital.

My surgery took place some 30 hours after admission—not bad by Canadian standards. I was fitted with an ankle brace and told to stay off my feet. Three weeks later I was Cleveland-bound, wheelchair and all. My flight from Vancouver to Toronto was relatively uneventful. I was loaded on board the airplane with a mobile board-chair device and had an aisle seat. The flight attendant only hit my cast boot once with the drink and food trolley! It is so great when people learn quickly.

The next issue was transferring from one terminal to another, which included a bus ride, en route to my Toronto-Cleveland airplane. This required the entire two-and-a-half-hour stopover. No problem, but it was now seven hours since I had been to a washroom to empty my bladder. Mercifully, both the flight and the Cleveland transport to my hotel were short. The bladder spasms were major and very frequent by then. It sounds like birth labour pains, doesn't it?! I checked in at the desk and made it to my room to go to the washroom, which was a considerable relief. There were more bladder spasms and then relative comfort. For the next three weeks, frequent voids and bladder spasms persisted.

New Perspectives

The MS symposium conference was amazing. I felt tickled pink and grateful to my MS Society Board of Directors for sending me as their representative. There were long presentations about MRI changes or non-changes relative to the "Big Three Drugs": Interferon beta-1a, Interferon beta-1b, and Glatimer Acetate. The speakers restated that it was still very difficult, if possible at all, to correlate clinical findings in an MS patient with MRI findings. This is perhaps where the individual's spirit, doggedness, or "control" of his or her own destiny steps in. In my near decade with MS, and my meeting of hundreds of MS people, this gap between clinical MRI and clinical status seems to persist.

At the MS symposium, coffee time or break time was a whole new issue for me. There were two wheelchairs and three scooters among some 400 participants. I have never been so invisible in my life! The experience changed my wheelchair perspective, for life. Nancy Holland, one of the major players in the U.S. MS Society, was helpful and instantly recognized my frustration. In addition, she made available two of the pending booklets on symptom management of MS complications.

These included bladder issues, pain issues, and fatigue. These booklets are a very useful algorithm or decision tree pattern for clinicians caring for MS patients. Those of us with MS should access these booklets from our local MS Society for our own knowledge and to share with our primary care physicians. Some neurologists will also benefit, as MS is sometimes a minor portion of their practice.

Information and knowledge are the kingpins to acquire if we are to optimally control our own destiny. This is especially key for those of us living in one of two "hinterlands," including rural and also dense, urban living. Ready access to an MS clinic will minimize this need, but access is not routinely available to many of us with MS. I realize a purist (e.g., MS neurologist) would like to have this information for only confirmed MS cases. However, after my own four years of Family Practice, where pre-diagnosis or pre-disease confirmation Is common, I know that we need to broaden our scope. I understand the average time to MS diagnosis is still six to seven years. These "waiting to be diagnosed" folks still deserve some symptom management, particularly with non-harmful or non-addicting therapeutic choices. This potential vacuum turns some people to go outside of regular channels, to seek more information, knowledge, and even solutions. Our hope is that this book can bridge the gap or at least temporize some of these issues. Certainly the waiting time and the frustration due to the lack of solutions make these individuals vulnerable to the many friends and neighbours with anecdotes galore. It may be these very different paths that stir the pot of frustration and mistrust between divergent groups. Knowledge, facts, and "do no harm" solutions can help resolve this disparity.

Now back to the conference, and time for me to get off my soapbox! The next important consideration is the network of people I met, including a gathering of Canadian MS Society representatives. We watched an excellent video that taught youngsters what MS in their parent might look like. For example, mittens simulated loss of touch and double-vision eyeglasses simulated vision problems encountered in MS. Of course, we all enjoyed an evening tour of the "Rock 'n' Roll" museum. Most of us could relate to the origins of Chubby Checker and Elvis Presley. My report of the conference to the Board spoke highly of the value of the networking, the forming of relationships, and the knowledge gleaned from the meeting. If this sort of activity interests you, get active in your MS Society!

One of the long-term goals of our Victoria, Canada–based MS Society has been easier accessibility to an MS clinic with MS neurologists and a multi-disciplinary team. Through the efforts of our MS Society Board in Victoria, the MS Clinic at UBC (University of British Columbia, Vancouver, BC), Dr. Joel Oger, and the MS-BC Division of MS Canada, this easier accessibility came to fruition. The clinic experienced growing pains, but all in all our efforts considerably improved the plight of people diagnosed with MS. This usually eliminated the two-hour ferry ride each way to and from Vancouver and the long, long day for a group of very low energy people and their caregivers.

But appointment time and space were almost immediately at a premium. The MS nurse was pulled in too many directions at once. Resolution was achieved when space was obtained by MS neurologist, Dr. Hrebicek, at the nearby Royal Jubilee Hospital in Victoria. The MS neurologist and MS nurse moved to the hospital scenario, closer to their pattern of practice and to that of most Canadian MS clinics. The two-year trial of a solely community-based facility shifted to today's workable hospital and community-based facility. I went from being extremely keen to have MS neurologists on site in the community to less so. I am now happy that the two are separate. It takes time for paradigm shifts to occur, and now I, too, am more patient. I would like to thank, publicly, all the people involved in the above process for their efforts. Vancouver Island (approximately 700,000 people, 1,300 of which are MS patients) has moved forward considerably in the last seven years. It is this island's "struggle with change" that has moved me, a specialty physician, to write this book.

In summary, my recommendation is that all of us diagnosed with MS should participate in a "newly diagnosed/newly accepting the diagnosis" group. I have added the "newly accepting" or "coming out about MS" as one step or stage in the healing process. In my experience, some of us take years to get to this stage. Perhaps it is like the four stages of grieving about death: anger, denial, grief, and acceptance. In no uncertain terms, chronic illness is a major turning point in life. Until we accept and recognize such a change, we cannot fully react to, respond to, or "heal" the problem. We are not an illness, but our illness is a component of who we are and how we embrace life thereafter. If we do not win this battle of wills, then our illness can and often does take over and get the upper hand.

By the way, an MS Society should exist in your community; if not, look around and start one. Ideally try to start one group for those who have had MS long term and another group for the "newly diagnosed" and/or "newly accepting" of a diagnosis. "Newly accepting" includes those "out of the closet," which can be 1-25 years. We all benefit from the sharing of each other's experiences, contacts, and networks. Many of us will not progress to walking assists or wheelchairs. Yet, the more we educate and understand each other, the more hope is possible. Certainly the bumps and knocks of our life experience are useful. Feelings of bitterness and hopelessness are temporary, so let's shorten them as quickly as possible.

CHAPTER TWELVE

Caregivers at Home and in the Community

S ignificant MS can dictate the need to receive and accept care. Denise and I have struggled with these issues, and my having been an official "caregiver" (as a physician family practice) made this issue even more clouded for us. My denial of MS worked all right for a time. However, once the "wake-up call" became loud and clear, I had to "get it" and stop work, which truly aggravated my lack of self-worth. Over the years, as a male, I had defined my self-worth by helping those in my personal reach and practice of medicine. With the onset of MS, my self-esteem plummeted. It took awhile to figure out how to build caregiving roles inside of our relationship. But we began the journey together and it took many turns, hit bottom, and soared as well.

Uncertainty

Fear and the uncertainty of what will happen in your life due to MS are major complications. We are all a combination of personal circumstances and interactions. If you meet others with MS for the first time at a long-established support group, most likely it will be a very negative and upsetting experience for you. Why? Because we incorrectly assume that if most of these people are wheelchair bound, or are having trouble walking, then we will too! I still remember medical school when we were exposed to difficult genetic syndromes for several hours a day, several days a week. What were my female classmates who were pregnant at that time thinking? "Will my baby be born with a birth defect?" It is very hard to keep our emotions and fears in a normal perspective when personal experience strongly suggests otherwise. The ultimate fear of severe MS, how it will burden the family or others, greatly challenges the caregiver. This is why we wanted to include a chapter on this important issue.

Women are more often the caregivers, just as they are more often the ones raising children. However, 70% of those with MS are women. This, too, is a great challenge on a relationship when "role reversal" becomes necessary. It also makes the sustaining or nurturing of the relationship with the caregiver incredibly important. Perhaps what we should be saying is that each caregiver and affected individual needs to take special steps to optimize or even survive his or her role. We believe adapting to this physical and economic change is a key piece of the acceptance and recovery puzzle. In the following discussion we hope to outline some of the components that have helped us.

Getting Help

First, when I was initially diagnosed, Denise's workplace had a modest but available Employee Assistance Program (EAP). This made several counseling sessions possible for us as a couple. Loss of job/health is one of life's greatest stresses and this counseling helped us verbalize and accept the change. We suggest that everyone seek out a similar option. As a self-employed physician, I did not have such an option. If there is no EAP, look for other types of support—such as your local MS Society, family services, or community groups such as a service club or church.

Second, we sought follow-up and received it from our Victoria-based MS Society. Our family met for 60-90 minutes with the Society's social worker to explore the impact my illness had on all five of us—Laura, Brian, Warren, Denise, and me. Laura, our youngest, had to change schools because of our financial crisis. She did this willingly, without whining, complaining, or fanfare. This was incredibly helpful to us. Our sons, Warren and Brian, were much more willing to help me out once they understood that my irritability and short fuse were MS-based.

Third, our local United Church minister followed our family closely with support during this time of crisis. For more than a year, I was listed weekly under "Prayers of Support." Now, we are both more able to understand the significance of "universal consciousness" and support—it is an important part of the healing possible in the "mind, body, and spirit" connection. Dr. Michael Greenwood discusses part of this in his book *Paradox of Healing.* In their books, Drs. Larry Dossey and Bernie Siegel also address the significance of prayer and caring.

Forgiveness

Our ability to accept our own trials and to forgive others—and to forgive ourselves—is very important. We hung on to anger for many months and still have some, years later. But, thankfully, we have been able to let it go for the most part. Some three years after, the person who was the source of my most painful interaction asked for my forgiveness before moving from our community. We attended the farewell for him and his wife, and although that occasion took considerable effort, it was a key part of acceptance and healing for both of us.

The fourth component that helped us was family caregiving. My mom and dad already lived quite close by when I became ill. They were very active in giving their time, energy, and even money when we were in sore need of all three. My parents' input and a very supportive personal bank manager meant we did not lose our home or emu farm. Then my dad was diagnosed with a lymphoma cancer six months after I was diagnosed with MS. This meant that I needed to give back to him after six months of accepting support from him. It also eased tension between all of us. Mom was now very committed to Dad's trials of radiation, chemotherapy, and finally his slow, reasonably comfortable death at home.

In addition, this pulled my brothers and sisters back together in common support of their parents. Our relationships had been very strained following our brother Stewart's death three years earlier. We believe all of us underestimate the power and significance of shared grief and circumstance.

Births and weddings are ready markers for us, as are deaths and other crises such as moving, job loss, or health loss. Certainly life continues on around us despite our illnesses.

Key Issues

Key issues for caregivers are support and respite. Bonnie, the social worker for our Victoria-based MS-Canada Society, always features the caregiver as a discussion topic in her eight sessions to help people share their ideas and frustrations and even exchange emails or phone numbers to build care networks. These discussions also build hope for the future, crucial for the caregiver as well. Whenever hope is lost, it is a huge task to regain it. People can climb mountains, but rarely do if we tell them it can't be done.

Key issues for caregivers are support and respite.

Respite is an opportunity for a break away from "constant" caring. The more continuous (i.e., 24-hour) care is required, the more critical is the need for frequent breaks for the caregiver. Many times family or friends supply coverage. However, often this is impossible or just not enough. Here again, support from your MS Society can be very helpful. The phrase "All you have to do is ask" needs to be emphasized over and over again. Usually it is just the pride of the MS patient or the caregiver that gets in the way. There is a country-western song that says, "It's my belief, pride is the chief cause of the decline of the number of husbands and wives." When one in a pair or family is stricken with chronic illness, this pride becomes a danger zone. Our ability to maintain close relationships, or reduce toxic ones, can have a profound influence on everyone's health. If the caregiver falters, or leaves, the patient frequently needs institutional care. In multiple sclerosis, this very rarely permits the return of independent living.

Denise's Story

Although we—Bill and Denise—have largely shared the writing of this journey so far, Denise wanted to add a personal note about her caregiving experiences:

The diagnosis of a chronic illness can put any person or family into a tailspin. How was I to know I was suddenly going to become a caregiver? Although I had worked in healthcare and had encountered many people facing a serious illness, I did not fully realize the ramifications in my own life. Personal experience is a great teacher. Initially, I was too numb to deal with the diagnosis. I concentrated my efforts on just making it through each day. Bill's moods were volatile. I think the emotional fallout of chronic illness is far more difficult to cope with than any physical changes that occur. Other caregivers dealing with family illness will no doubt identify with this.

In truth, I cannot recall many of the details of the first three years of Bill's illness. It was like I had plummeted down a black hole of despair. Bill was so sick and I felt there was not much I could do to make him better. I do know that I was angry and fearful, both destructive emotions. I was angry at an illness that took away Bill's ability to do work at which he was so very talented. I was angry at an illness that had come at a time in our lives that was happy and good. I could not understand the "why" behind the illness.

I was fearful of our now unknown future. As Bill's symptoms worsened, I was fearful that he would lose his independence and become more disabled. Would I lose my husband, my soul mate? We were supposed to grow old together, enjoying our children as adults and grandchildren to come. It seemed as though our social life had been reduced to people in wheelchairs, people who were becoming more and more disabled by this dreadful disease. I was fearful, as the bills accumulated, and no money came in, that we would lose our home. I was also worried about the impact on our three children. They had experienced Bill's mood swings and knew too well the tension in the household.

I am glad that I persevered; I am glad that I weathered the storm. I am grateful that our children have also "hung in there." Gradually, as time passed, Bill seemed to get a bit better. The chaos settled down. The stress levels declined. It seemed like we were emerging from the long, dark tunnel. We began to socialize more and didn't feel like we were in "survival mode" only. It became possible to envision a future again.

What we experienced individually, and as a family, is no doubt similar to what many experience when a chronic or life-threatening illness strikes. Some of the things I found very helpful were the counseling sessions that Bill previously mentioned. These sessions gave me an opportunity to vent my anger and fears in a safe environment. I would encourage anyone struggling with illness and disability to seek help from a professional counselor. Church affiliation was extremely beneficial. The visits from people in our church and from our minister were very much appreciated, as were their prayers. Support and assistance from friends was also appreciated. I am part of a women's group that meets to share stories and songs. I am grateful for the listening ears and compassionate support from this group.

I am also extremely grateful for the support provided by Bill's parents. The help they provided, in so many ways, was invaluable. We feel blessed by the support and understanding of our three children. Without the love and support from these and other family members, it would have been so much more difficult.

When reflecting back on the past few years, many thoughts come to mind. One is the importance of relationships, be they with family, friends, or the people we associate with in church, at the gym, in service clubs, or other types of groups. When the going gets tough, the support from these sources can make a big difference.

Another realization is the importance of support groups such as the MS Support Group that Bill has been involved in and of umbrella organizations such as the MS Society of British Columbia as well as local chapters. So much good work is being done with fairly limited funds. Bill and I have supported these groups over the years since his diagnosis and we look forward to continued involvement. So, if a critical illness strikes your family, seek out the local support groups. You will all benefit greatly.

Another reflection is the unpredictability of life and the ability to trust in a Higher Power. For a long time, I could not grasp why this was happening to us. I now believe that many things happen in life that are not within our control, but are being orchestrated by a Higher Power. There are no coincidences in life. Bill's destiny was not to be an anesthetist; rather, his medical training and skills have prepared him for the work he does now in educating others with chronic illness. He not only offers helpful advice, but he also provides people with hope for better health. Nor was my destiny to remain within traditional healthcare. I feel that my contribution now complements Bill's work and also benefits people in ways I could not have otherwise achieved. The world is full of endless opportunity—we look forward to the future with great optimism. We all need to trust that things will work out over time. Helen Keller's words seem especially appropriate: "When a door of happiness closes, another opens; but often we look so long at the closed door that we do not see the one which has been opened for us."

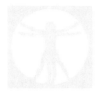

CHAPTER THIRTEEN

Financial Challenges and Solutions

This topic will be very significant to many of you with MS who face job loss, interruptions, or reduced working hours. The likelihood of recovery is reduced if you feel trapped by finances, bills, and phone hassles with creditors. We know this only too well as we hit the wall and were juggling bank overdrafts with credit card upper limits month after month. Financial issues were a major part of the illness crisis for us. We very nearly lost everything when the illness ended my anesthesiology practice, despite having a sizable income before diagnosis. Our savings (RRSPs in Canada or IRAs in the United States) went to paying acute debt (deferred taxes and emu farm expenses), and we worried that despite all our hard work and years of training we would be penniless.

Loss of a primary relationship through death or divorce is all too common in MS or any major chronic illness. Each of us must seek all the help we can in this tough, one- to two-year period when we progress from relapsing-remitting MS to secondary MS, or when we start with primary progressive MS. An MS expert at Scripps Clinic in San Diego, California, diagnosed me with primary progressive MS. In reality, once you reach the progressive stage, it matters little whether it is primary or secondary MS. Treatments by traditional medicine are quite limited, with symptom management, or control, the best they can do.

It is in this respect that we believe the individual or couple has to be especially proactive. We all need to feel empowered, to feel that we can control our own destiny. Without hope, deterioration can be rapid, severe, and lead to depression or institutionalization. In our experience, most people diagnosed with a significant degree of MS will need to reduce their working hours or quit their job.

Bureaucracy Challenges

The road to financial stability in MS can be rocky and tortuous. Bureaucracy is tough to deal with when you are physically and mentally exhausted. The recurrent insurance forms still need to be carefully and meticulously done. Try to make it a game; if you take it too personally, the bureaucracy wins. Most disability programs are full of detail and repetition, which causes frustration. Our advice is to get the very best guidance and information you can. Often this means linking up with your local MS Society or chapter. We had considerable problems with the application for disability in spite of my time in family medicine practice as well as having a conscientious and experienced family practitioner, Dr. Candace Cole. The bureaucracy pushed us to the limit, including nearly two years of waiting. In addition, we were finally advised that our case needed to be heard by a "tribunal" for a final decision and it was difficult to find "team support." After four months, one week before the scheduled tribunal, they relented and agreed that we qualified for a disability pension. (In retrospect, we wish we had looked for help sooner through our Vancouver Island MS chapter, part of the MS Society of British Columbia, and part of MS Canada. You, too, will have a local, state/provincial, or national body near you. It is up to you to seek their help, online, in person, or any other way you can. This is one service at which they are good, because of their experience. You need their help. So—ask for it!)

The following are useful concepts anyone with MS should consider when applying for disability benefits:

1. Look for allies—those who have expertise in your community, one of the MS support groups, or even the government. Your local MS Society, especially a social worker there, can point you in a good direction. Our

extremely supportive lawyer colleague wisely says, "Don't let those bastards grind you down, 'cause that's what they want to do!" In fact, bureaucrats are often rewarded for keeping or getting you off a disability payroll. Keep your long-term needs in mind and take it one step at a time.

2. Complete insurance or disability forms only when you are in your clearest thinking state. We have been supremely appreciative of the assistance of friends and their associates in this matter. If you quit on your valid disability application, then the bureaucrats win! The insurance companies would rather not pay out money. One to two years of economic hardship can turn into a decade, even a lifetime.

3. Positive work and income options are needed. If you are fortunate, you may be able to develop an ongoing, flexible relationship with your workplace. Beware of inner pride! Some of us with MS will not "take advantage of" or "abuse" our disability. Please give your head a shake. Being diagnosed with MS is a life-altering experience. Acceptance of your diagnosis and taking control of your work, diet, and exercise empowers you to make the best of your situation. Pride and the fear of "being treated with pity" are dangerous defense mechanisms. Take pride in what you can do, whether exercise, grooming, or listening to a friend. Taking pride in your "closet MS" secret is dangerous and can work to your long-term detriment. Denial of MS is no more useful than denial of a cancer diagnosis.

Earning Income

What options do you have regarding earning income? Usually you will need to plug into a network of business associates or friends who still value your input. I was fortunate to eventually become the "world's expert" on emu oil. This gave me some self-esteem and made me feel needed again. We need to find a niche for our passion or expertise. Think long and hard about this issue. Home-based businesses are more available today than ever before.

Today, Denise and I are passionate about educating and empowering people to eat right and be aware of the food supplements that are optimal for health. Fulfilling a niche as an educator is often possible. Distributing health or wealth information, tutoring, and even direct sales are all niches for educators. The Internet is a new cornerstone for this option. Coupled with low telephone rates, it increases our options of working solely, or at least part time, from home.

Consider your own knowledge and skills. We are all now in the "information age." This creates a new business niche called "information entrepreneurs" or to use Robert Allan's term "infopreneurs." This book is an example of our moving into this infopreneurial stage. Our goal is to provide up-to-date health information for people with MS or other chronic illnesses. Chronic illness is increasing in many parts of the industrialized world. This book is an important building block in our long-term financial security.

My being diagnosed with MS has changed my perspective greatly. Flexibility and diversification are key. We have taken many personal development and training courses, most recently with Mark Victor Hansen, known for the *Chicken Soup for the Soul* series. (See *Appendix A & B* for Internet links.) Books, community resources, disability resource groups, and even MS chapters will enhance your awareness of options. Yes, you may be forced to create your own employment, so make it one you like!

Home-Based Businesses

Certainly many of today's products are first available through direct sales, Internet, mail order, or networking companies. This makes sense, no matter whether it is a special food supplement, book, newsletter, or healthcare product. This allows the client the option to "shop" or "sell" from home. These features dovetail well with many of us who are relatively community- or homebound individuals. We believe this is particularly important for young, single parents, who are primarily women in their 20s, 30s, and 40s when MS peaks. So, please, go to our website, not just to buy something, but also for ideas "outside the box," where you could work with us or for us, or even emulate what we are doing. If the Internet is not an option for you, send us a letter or telephone us, using the contact information listed under *Resources*.

Again, we firmly believe a home-based business can be a valuable option for many. What are some of the advantages of a home-based business? First, many costs can be minimized. Second, some of your costs, such as office space, computers, utilities, telephone, Internet, car, and even clothing (especially dry cleaning) may be tax deductible, from earned or even other income. In Canada, for example, often $6,000-8,000 per year may be reasonable to deduct from your "other" salary income, before paying your income tax.

We first did this with our emu hobby farm project. Denise was on salary as a dietician, and this side, home-based business helped reduce her tax bite. In fact, in Canada, you can barely afford not to have a home-based business, for this reason alone. The major requirement is that you must have reasonable expectation of profit within two years of start-up. I have watched vineyards and Christmas tree farms spin this out over seven or eight years.

Third, start-up costs are usually reasonable. A package or business start-up kit is often available and can be acquired for less than $1,000. Another business option is a franchise, or ready-to-go "cookie cutter" business. This, often, is considerably more expensive. Do your due diligence. Talk to friends or people you trust who can help you with this.

Certainly our last three years of education, training, and hands-on experience have allowed us considerable expertise in this area. Health information and health products can be lucrative businesses as we baby boomers (born 1945-1966) age and move toward retirement. Most of us are seriously looking at staying healthy. Your venturing into this sphere can be as simple as joining our team by purchasing a health product that you respect or simply want to try. As with most things, you should first try a product. If it helps you, you are on your way toward success, as your personal story will mean a great deal to others. Personal care and beauty products have been successfully promoted in this manner; consider Avon or Mary Kay cosmetics.

We are most happy within health products. This encompasses our passions, our expertise, and now our successful personal story of recovery for each of us. We need new team players with us, in all regards. Our experience with most people with MS is that they have a zest for life and are great people for getting things done. Movers and shakers, regardless of individual disability, are people we can work with. Your first step in due diligence might be as simple as listening to us speak, meeting us personally, or even via mail, telephone contact, or email. Now is the perfect time for a home-based business to interact with others, even across long distances or globally.

Our wealth information training has taught us to work toward multiple streams of passive income. This could be as simple as a network marketing affiliation, owning a car wash or laundromat, or as complex as an ongoing newsletter and book on your expertise or passion. One example we recall hearing was of a man with 20 years experience in selling and repairing refrigerators. He started an evening seminar on fridges to teach homeowners the nuances of what was available, and what might work best for them, their kitchen, and their lifestyle. Subsequently, he became the number one fridge salesman and entrepreneur in that city or region. Another success story is a woman from Saskatchewan who solved a problem and then sold the solution. Her observation was that many newborn calves had their ears frozen during Canadian winters. Her "ear muffs for calves" became very popular among cattle ranchers and farmers alike!

Network Marketing

Network marketing, especially with a unique or excellent product, has matured over the last three decades. In the 1960s, it meant buying and then selling a garage-full of soap. Then, in the 1970s and '80s, it became a personal trust and relationship business for home and personal care products.

By the 1990s and to date, this has matured further, with health and well-ness products. The Internet and inexpensive telephone and travel have permitted this burgeoning health and wellness industry to add unique prod-ucts that require some education by experts. An example of this is the envelope of whey protein isolate described in this book.

In today's world, network marketing or direct sales has many advan-tages. Besides low start-up costs, the people handling the sales (i.e., distributors) do not have to buy or carry an inventory of product. Instead, the distributor assists the customer in accessing product from the company, usually by use of a credit card. The product is then shipped directly to the customer's residence. The distributor is then responsible for follow-up with the customer. Income for the distributor is based on the volume of product purchased by customers. Income is also generated when the distributor recruits other people who become distributors. Communication today is fast and easy with the use of machines, cell phones, computers, conference calls, 3-way calls, and couriers.

An important advantage of network marketing is the ability to gener-ate more income than a regular job might provide. Hard work and building relationships can pay off in direct sales. Furthermore, network marketing allows for the leverage of time and the generation of a passive income. "Passive income" means income that is generated even when you do not actively work the business. Passive income occurs as a result of training oth-ers to do the job (duplication).

Another significant advantage of a credible, successful, well-estab-lished direct sales company is training. The men and women who work as independent distributors within these companies can train you. Corporate training is often available as well. We still prefer the one-on-one or "kitchen meeting" training. This is people interaction at its best—problem solving, networking, and emotional sharing of wisdom. Two of our best friends, Frank and Paul, came to us because of our involvement in a direct sales company. We mention this because men rarely develop close friends with other males, and they need this every bit as much as women do.

Finally, in our era of big box stores providing many of our personal needs, there are still times we would like to speak or interact with a real person. If that direct sales or network marketing individual has developed trust in his or her relationships, and maintains that trust, it becomes a win-win situation. Furthermore, if one or more members of that individual's team has a high degree of credibility, that success or business opportunity is further enhanced. We agree that women are better as network entrepreneurs. However, any of us can succeed if we develop trust and follow with our interpersonal skills rather than the "hard sell"—often thought of, but now outdated.

If work in your regular area of employment is not possible because of MS, or if network marketing, infopreneurship, or other types of work are not options, then perhaps volunteering is. Many of us with MS volunteer our time, energy, and wisdom to help others with MS or other life challenges. Scan your community for options to volunteer. There are many service clubs and nonprofit organizations that are eager for help. Being a volunteer can be rewarding. Not only will you have the opportunity to discover new friends or develop new skills, but you will also benefit spiritually—helping others is good for the soul!

In summary, a number of potential courses of action exist, despite a life-altering illness. Be creative, sincere, and, if need be, humble in looking for new solutions. Often volunteering in something you enjoy or believe in can be a great start. Similarly, if family or others offer to help, then create a way they can. This benefits both of you in the long term—health-wise and/or financially. Learn all you can about your disability options, regarding pensions or tax deductions. Remember, knowledge is power. Finally, begin today, step-by-step, to create a new personal network. Any steps you take will enhance your chances of recovery in mind, body, and spirit.

CHAPTER FOURTEEN

Sexuality and Bladder Issues

The changes that take place in our bodies, secondary to MS, are quite varied. Some of the earliest changes may often involve the bladder and perineal/genital area. Once it is determined that we have MS, many of us can look back on the changes in our bladder patterns as being an often ongoing, persistent problem that we had tried to explain to ourselves in some other way. I recall having troubles voiding (the emptying of all or part of the bladder), particularly while standing, for 10-15 years prior to diagnosis. I falsely assumed that I must have had an early prostate partial blockage of the bladder outflow tract. My adaptation: sitting down to empty my bladder. Hesitancy in starting voiding is common in MS.

Bladder Issues

The most likely reason for early and/or persistent bladder changes is our anatomy. The nerve supply to the bladder and sexual organs has long and relatively small nerves running lengthwise from the brain to the lowest part of the spine. (The medical term is *cranio-sacral outflow of the parasympathetic pathway*.) These very long, small nerve tracts are quite likely to be more susceptible to early "injury" by MS "attacks" or demyelination.

Bladder symptoms for men and women include more frequent voidings. The incomplete emptying of the bladder creates a place in which bacteria can grow—frequently resulting in bladder infections. This is especially likely in women, as the urethra (tube from bladder to outside) is particularly short (1-2 cm in women compared to 10-15 cm in men). This short distance makes the female bladder especially vulnerable to infections, particularly E. coli bacteria, a common component of our bowel tract and feces (hence the importance for women of wiping front to back and wearing cotton panties to prevent bladder infections). Women are also at risk for "honeymoon cystitis," that is, bladder infection following frequent intercourse. "Honeymoon cystitis" is believed to be due to the "friction" or rubbing of intercourse, which can inflame the urethral opening, making it more susceptible to bacterial infection. Emptying the bladder within 30-60 minutes of having intercourse can minimize these infections.

The incomplete emptying of the bladder creates a place in which bacteria can grow–frequently resulting in bladder infections.

MS folks are more prone to bladder infection because the MS changes in the nerve supply cause incomplete emptying of the bladder. This residual urine is unfortunately a "sitting duck" for infection. Urine contains warm water and protein, both of which are needed for rapid bacterial growth. In the past, residual urine could only be determined by in-and-out catheterization. Now a bladder ultrasound (similar to the one taken during pregnancy) is simple and non-invasive.

In 1998 I developed a bladder infection due to preoperative catheterization prior to the repair of my badly fractured ankle. The Vancouver –Toronto–Cleveland flight was a huge challenge for me. After a two-week trip involving many cramps, urgencies, and some sweats, a course of antibiotics quickly resolved the problem.

This was an honest mistake, but points to the need for a high index of suspicion when dealing with bladder infections, especially in women with MS. Early diagnosis and treatment relieves many symptoms, but will also reduce your risk of the infection spreading "upriver" to the kidneys. We believe regular, pure cranberry juice, dried cranberries, or cranberry capsules are a useful assist for women with MS. Why? Because it has been documented that the cranberry reduces the likelihood of E. coli bacteria "implanting," or taking up residence, in the bladder wall. We recommend pure cranberry juice rather than the heavily sweetened cranberry cocktail. New data suggests that blueberries are as effective as cranberries for bladder health. If these simple steps are inadequate, then visit your physician for medical advice.

MS folks are more prone to bladder infection because the MS changes in the nerve supply cause incomplete emptying of the bladder.

My relationship with a bright, well-trained urologist in our city, Dr. Bill Nielsen, permitted one other useful nugget in bladder troubles. Saw palmetto, by mouth, affects bladder receptors. Until recently, healthcare practitioners felt it worked on slowing prostate enlargement and, hence, only in men. We now know a quality saw palmetto soothes some of the key irritable bladder receptors. It is these irritated receptors that trigger those of us with MS to get up several times a night. For this we recommend taking 15 ml or 1 tablespoon daily of a Canadian-researched, quality saw palmetto. (See *Appendix A & B.*) This limits me to one bathroom wake-up call per night, and several women with MS have also much improved their sleep pattern by using this liquid, available without prescription.

Sexuality Issues

Now I'd like to speak intimately about the sexual changes of MS, which I've been skirting long enough! The early sensory changes, particularly in the genital area, often complicate sex in many ways. In women, the very sensitive skin and mucosal surfaces of the vulva, labia, and vaginal entrance, or clitoris, can send mixed messages to both partners. This hypersensitivity can actually be painful, reducing the usual lubrication of foreplay

and diminishing coital pleasure, or eliminating it altogether. This is particularly troubling to a young couple where one of the pair has MS. The
importance of caring, frank, and patient discussion between the couple cannot be overstated. The changes in our lovemaking due to my MS occurred
20 years into our marriage. These types of changes usually occur earlier in
women, as MS often begins in women in the late teens, 20s, and 30s.

Sexuality and, more importantly, intimacy are key components of a
lasting relationship. And relationships are a very important part of our mind-
body-spirit continuum. A healthy body, mind, and spirit are essential to our
well-being, and to our recovery from and control of MS. Any resource—
whether counseling, education, or even a weekend or longer away for the
couple—is valuable.

Relationships are one of the most volatile issues for MS folks. When
my health was rapidly spiraling downhill, I tried to push Denise away. I
thought I was worthless and that I was on my way to the pit of despair or
institutionalization. Even worse, I was worried that I would be a huge draw
on our family's meager economic resources. But Denise was stubborn. She
didn't budge. She was in our relationship for the long haul. This was incredibly important to me.

Over the last five to six years, our lovemaking has needed to adapt
and transcend the hectic lifestyle trials and tribulations of Denise's work
and our three children. The brain-erection connection has been virtually
severed for me. This means local area touching and stroking is essential
for erection to occur. Also, frequent feedback between the couple of
what feels good, and what does not, is very important. This "brain-erection connection" change means I can no longer tell whether I have an
erection or not without seeing or hand-checking. Similarly, I cannot usually tell if I am inside the vagina or not. Happily, the pleasures of touch
and ejaculation are still in place. Similar situations happen to many
people with MS, in different ways.

These changes are often aggravated by the "mind numbing" fatigue of
MS. The MS individual is often "too tired" to even be interested in sex.

I believe "the invisible" fatigue is perhaps the most common and generally debilitating symptom of MS, as it occurs in 85% of us. Severe fatigue hampers MS folks' ability to adapt well to the change or loss of their senses, mobility, or strength. Adaptation to change is a large component of what makes us human. For some years MS fatigue limited communication between Denise and me. Fatigue also left me feeling like a "naked nerve ending," which hampered intimacy between us. Reversal of fatigue has helped both of us, and our relationship, to progress forward to new levels of growth, trust, and self-esteem.

Suggested Solutions:

1. Warm or even tepid baths, together with Epsom salts, magnesium sulfate (bath salts), and aromatherapy. This time of relaxation, enhanced by aromatherapy (e.g., lavender), will help intimacy to proceed. See Chapter 17 on the five senses for charts on aroma therapy. (Also see *Appendix A & B*.)

2. Use of erotic oils for one or both partners. Emu oil will lower pain hypersensitivity. (See *Appendix A & B*.)

3. Time together away from the hectic world in peaceful, serene settings, best near nature!

Number 1. will tend to reduce the nerve irritability of MS and perhaps muscle spasms as well. The joint comfort product listed in *Resources* is very helpful at reducing muscle pain and spasms, too. An important reminder, is to not put the joint comfort on mucous membranes such as eyes or genital surfaces, the hands should be washed after use.

Before completing this chapter, I want to include our suggestions for those with advanced MS—particularly relating to the bladder and sex. If MS progresses, catheterization may at some point be required. In my travels around North America, I learned of a patented and FDA-approved device with a special valve that helps pool and intermittently flush out urine from the bladder. This more closely approximates the filling of a normal, full bladder and then the complete emptying of this greater volume. Similarly, it may reduce bladder infections by the "flushing" of this temporarily stored urine. It may help minimize bladder spasms as well. If the bladder can still fill somewhat, sexual intercourse can be made more normal, as well, by temporarily removing the catheter. One other option many of us do not know about is the supra pubic (above the pelvic bone) catheter. Ask your urologist if and when this would be a useful option.

Finally, many of the foregoing suggestions may reduce bladder infection, the bane of many MS folks' existence. Similarly, the enhanced cell-mediated immunity of our white blood cells, from increasing glutathione in the body, may reduce the frequency of antibiotics being required. See Chapter 4 on glutathione (GSH) and its role in preventing infection. This is quite important, as many of us become either sensitized (allergic) or develop bacterial resistance to these antibiotics.

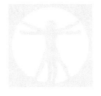

CHAPTER FIFTEEN

Walking, Balance, and Nerve Pathway Retraining

L oss of mobility, whether it is walking or using one's arms, is frequently encountered in MS. In our observation and experience, the inability to walk has two contributing factors. Loss of balance, or proprioception, is often a problem. Secondarily, loss of muscle strength aggravates the balance Issue. Folks with MS will state one or the other, or both, as walking/mobility issues.

Let us start with what is perhaps the easiest to explain. In almost all cases, the muscles and the nerves that supply them are fine. We must remember, however, that when a body tissue or pathway is unused it starts to fade or become ineffective. The motor nerve simply leaves the spinal cord and arrives at the muscle. But we need to understand that even though we started with some 250 muscles at birth, by our 30s we are down to 80, even as low as 50. Why such a difference? If you don't use it you lose it! This includes many of our less or almost never used muscles, such as the ones that act as stabilizers for our standing and walking, and the fine-tuning muscles, such as the ones that pull our thighs together (adductors) or apart (abductors).

When any of our "walking" muscles are deprived of their nerve supply in our spinal cord or brain, that muscle use is diminished or even lost completely. Subsequently, the body quickly learns a new "gait" or way of walking that is almost always abnormal and not efficient. It skews our walking, disturbs our balance, and even affects some of our joints as well. We credit Meir Schneider, of California, for first introducing this to us, and credit some of our MS friends for reinforcing it. He was legally blind until 17 years of age before learning that he could recruit or retrain "backup" motor nerve pathways. These are small eye muscles that control the eye's movement and "pair" the two eyes' movement to avoid "double vision." Vision loss and double vision are common symptoms in MS and can often be minimized by "balancing" and "low light training of the eye." Schneider was able to recover a considerable amount of his vision, which permitted a much more normal life, with improved, though not perfect, vision.

Backup Reserves

The concept that Meir Schneider presented to us, first in Vancouver, and then later in Victoria, was that our body possesses the great feature of redundancy, or "backup" or "reserve" motor nerves. This means that the specialized motor nerve that is so important in balance and eye-hand coordination (i.e., proprioception) also has backup nerves that can be recruited to perform the same function. Another example would be the common belief regarding stroke recovery: that whatever abilities a person gains back in the first two years following a stroke will be the only ones he or she will *ever* gain back. But now we know that there are "spare" pathways we can train. Also, the younger you are when you receive a brain injury, the better your chances of a full recovery. This holds true for injuries to the spinal cord as well. In fact, you can remove one-half of the brain of a newborn and he or she can develop completely normal!

Our body possesses the great feature of redundancy, or "backup" or "reserve" motor nerves.

New concepts about our brain and spinal cord continue to emerge. The 1990s was the "decade of the brain" in the research world, and many contributions have shaken "old" ideas. For example, we only use an average of 10% of our brain during our lifetime. We suggest that some of us are not even using that 10% yet! Are we saving it?! This concept is incredibly important to those of us with a brain illness such as MS or who have had a traumatic injury. We now know we should never give up or abandon hope of recovery.

Eva Marsh, the Canadian who wrote *Black Patent Shoes, Dancing with MS*, has been a great inspiration to me. Though paralyzed a number of times with MS, she is still walking. Her education and research about the nervous system convinced her of this possibility. In fact, with the help of her two very young daughters, she recovered from one of her bouts of almost total paralysis. It wasn't easy but it certainly was worth all the trouble, because regaining independence is invaluable. She describes her brain's MRI (magnetic resonance imaging) as being a near

We know that there are "spare" pathways we can train.

whiteout. Apparently, when it is shown to neurologists, most of them ask how many years she has been in a wheelchair—but she is not!

Another point of note here is that your MRI is not necessarily consistent with your disability. What this means is a "bad" looking MRI may be an MRI of a fairly normal, well-functioning individual with MS. The converse is also true. The biggest determinant of your outcome, or recovery, is the "dedication" or "effort" you put into this body-mind-spirit scenario. The best example is people who have had a stroke and have lost the ability to speak. Almost always, if they work at it, they can recover their speech. It may be as tough or even harder than the first time they learned to speak, but it can be done. They regain their speech, not because they have retrained the injured piece of brain or the piece of brain has healed, but rather because they have trained or "recruited" a completely new part of the brain.

A further useful piece of knowledge we received recently from a woman with master's degrees in Speech Therapy and Voice (i.e., singing) pertained to the speech problems of people with MS. Her impression, with 20 years of experience behind it, is that most folks with MS have reduced power and quality of speech due to inadequate breathing techniques. She has seen great improvement in her own clients with Parkinson's disease. These methods of breathing can often be learned from voice/choir teachers in your own community. Better yet, a group or choir holds great benefits for the body, mind, and spiritual growth and for new relationships as well. I find singing tenor in a choir a valuable component of my health and spiritual journey. Practicing music, whether voice or an instrument (e.g., keyboard, guitar, or harp), is another great "recovery" or "nerve recruitment" method.

One other tip given to us by a wise physiotherapist specializing in MS is worth mentioning. If one of us with MS has a foot drop, but is not yet ready to accept a heel splint, there is another option. Buy a pair of lace-up boots, such as Roper boots or "granny" boots. The lace-up support worked for me for the three years until I was able to retrain those muscles.

Balance Challenges

Our awareness of where our body parts are enables us to stand, walk upright, and all variations thereof. In MS we frequently lose this balance and become almost completely dependent on our visual cues. This is the basis of the Romberg test, given to us by our physicians. In this we stand with our feet together, bare or stocking feet, hold our arms out in front of us and are asked to close our eyes. If we have MS, most often we will start to fall. Without our visual cues, we cannot sense where our body parts are. In addition, those with reduced vision or "double" or blurred vision from MS are further challenged when standing or walking. Wisely, we should reach for a cane or walker to achieve a more stable, three-pointed stance. These issues are further compounded by muscle weakness, whether from muscle disuse or vitamin D deficiency (see Chapter 5 on vitamin D). Again, our muscles are a "use it or lose it" proposition, hence the value of exercise.

How can we improve our proprioception, that is, our awareness of where our body parts are? Happily these nerve pathways are miniature motor nerve pathways, which means that the information centers are spread across our muscles (via gamma efferent fibers). When a muscle moves, these miniature motor nerve pathways send quick, tiny bits of information to the brain as the muscle contracts. This message to the brain is then coordinated with outgoing messages along nerves to smoothly move the muscle. Hence, if the major motor nerve pathway, let's call it #1 of 5, is interrupted in the spinal cord and/or brain, then the muscle does not move on command. Similarly, the miniature motor nerves that sense the position of the muscle are also interrupted. We perceive that we now have both less muscle strength and less awareness of where that muscle and body part is. These changes are why MS people often do badly on the Romberg test (standing with eyes closed) and finger-nose pointing test. Our eyes take on the extra job of telling us where all our body parts are. As soon as our eyes are closed, we do poorly.

The perfect way to send much more mini-muscle traffic or pathway information to the brain is to exercise in front of the mirror.

The perfect way to send much more mini-muscle traffic or pathway information to the brain is to exercise in front of the mirror. Move your arms slowly enough so your brain can retrain or recruit a group of new motor nerve position sense pathways. Here we use our eyes and muscle movement to retrain our position sense. An excellent lower limb recruitment method is to hold on to a chair, or something that is stable, then, while standing, lift one foot off the floor. Initially this is best done in front of a mirror, so that you can use your eyes to help. The more frequently we do this, moving our muscles through this range ourselves, or with an assistant, the more traffic we send to and from the brain and the quicker we will recruit new pathways. Similarly, even thinking about this adds more traffic. Now you can work at recruitment or retraining wherever and whenever you wish.

Connect, Connect, Connect with Others

Finally, we all do better working in teams or pairs. As human beings, we all crave attention and support for our efforts. So, join your local yoga, exercise facility, MS support group, or any similar group. Our local MS support group helped organize and subsidize yoga and tai chi for its members. Most MS support groups are part of MS chapters, which are affiliated with a region, state, province, or national MS Society. Please look at the discussion on MS organizations because these have been a key component of my own healing journey.

Each of us tends to identify with different heroes or we try to model ourselves after someone we trust and respect. To this end, we will now outline some people who have achieved a great deal despite having MS. Montel Williams is one of our favorite, physically active, MS people. His books are full of sensible, practical, and achievable goals. Similarly, his talk show regularly displays empathy, trust, and hope. Each of these is important in our own relationships and is necessary on our roadway to recovery. One of Montel's most recent books is *Body Change: The 21-Day Fitness Program for Changing Your Body ... and Changing Your Life!* This book was written in conjunction with his personal trainer, Wini Linguvic. The exercise routine incorporates aerobics, weight training, and core and functional exercises to improve your balance, coordination, and strength. We cannot think of a better approach than the one taken by Montel. Happily, this "Body Change Program" relies less on big, complex machines and more on free weights, a bench, and core exercises. The authors are accurate in calling their aerobics and weight training exercises "straightforward." However, they also ask, "What about

> *Rest or "energy management" is a useful coping skill. However, physical use of our body, in a safe venue, is one of the best and most important components in recovery.*

attitude?" Each of us must personally grab on to a new motivation to improve ourselves. Montel and Wini hope that in reading about their efforts to surmount challenges on the road to keeping fit or returning to fitness, we will see whatever excuse we have for not training or not training harder for exactly what it is—an excuse.

Many of our family and friends want us to rest, in order to speed our recovery. Now, after eight years with MS, we believe "rest" does not offer the benefit we thought it did. Rest or "energy management" is a useful coping skill. However, physical use of our body, in a safe venue, is one of the best and most important components in recovery. Certainly, a 21-day program may not fit with your capabilities at present. Why not a 42-, 63-, or 84-day program then? There is an incredible number of choices for us to follow and each one begins with a single step down that path.

A second individual's story that means a great deal to me and Denise is that of Meir Schneider, of San Francisco. We described his considerable recovery of sight due to recruitment of backup nerve pathways. When I first met him at the Vancouver Complementary Medicine seminar in 1997, he outlined his concepts. At that time, I was relatively mobile, but dragged my right foot and was reasonably weak on my right side. Meir had us slowly rotate our neck, first one way and then another, and note how much flexibility we had. Then he asked us to do a series of exercises with our hands and feet (shoes off). He showed us the much-improved flexibility in our neck, which occurred as the result of using our hands and feet! Meir was able to convince most people in the room how interconnected our nervous and muscle systems are.

We learned more from him a year or so later at another conference hosted by the MS Society of British Columbia, Capital Region Chapter in Victoria. Since that time, we have read his books and watched his video. A young woman with significant MS, who had walking problems, went to San Francisco to study under him. What she learned was a major part of her being able to walk normally again.

Start Moving Again

Many resources are available to us for beginning our walking recovery or long-term maintenance. One of our favorite teachers is Brenda Adam-Smith, a physiotherapist with Feldenkrais training who works for MS Canada, Capital Region Chapter, here in Victoria, B.C.

Her knowledge and study of new concepts, whether from the Alexander Technique, Meir Schneider's, or others, suggests that the originator of these concepts is Dr. Moshe Feldenkrais, DSc (1904-1984). We would like to tell you part of Dr. Feldenkrais' story as a tribute to his incredible contribution to those of us with MS or other CNS injuries (including stroke, cerebral palsy, or back pain), muscle injuries or illnesses. To begin this wonderful story, we will refer you to two books written by Feldenkrais' students. The first is *Awareness Heals: The Feldenkrais Method for Dynamic Health* by Steve Shafarman. The second is *Relaxercise: The Easy New Way to Health and Fitness* by David Zemach-Bersin, Kaethe Zemach-Bersin, and Mark Reese. These are excellent resources and are where I learned most of the Feldenkrais story. The original book by Moshe Feldenkrais is *Awareness through Movement* (Harper & Row, 1972). In simple, concrete terms, the Feldenkrais Method (FM) eliminates any division between body and mind. With the FM you can begin to live in ways that minimize or eliminate many problems. Steve Shafarman's book uses simple, common movements: bending, turning, leaning, breathing, sitting, and walking.

The Feldenkrais Method has a fascinating background. Moshe Feldenkrais was born in the Ukraine in 1904 and left home at the age of 14 to travel to Palestine mostly by foot. As a young man he studied in Tel Aviv, worked as a tutor, labourer, and surveyor. He loved sports, particularly soccer, a game in which he severely injured the ligaments and cartilage of his left knee. In 1928, he moved to Paris to study physics, math, and mechanical and electrical engineering. He went on to be principal assistant to Joliot-Courier (winner of 1935 Nobel Prize in Chemistry). While in Paris, he met Jigoro Kano, the developer of modern judo, and became one of the first Europeans to earn a black belt in judo.

In 1940, Moshe Feldenkrais escaped the Nazis by reaching England. He worked for the British Admiralty during World War II, helping to develop sonar and submarine detection. His wife, Yona Rubenstein, was a pediatrician. Throughout those years in his wife's office, he became very interested in human development, in children's movement, and especially in the movement of babies.

A bus accident aggravated his soccer knee injury. Surgeons offered only a 50% chance of recovery, so he went his own way. In pursuit of a better answer, he studied everything that was then known about health and healing. This included anatomy and physiology, neuro-physiology, exercise and movement therapies, psychotherapy and spiritual practices, yoga, hypnosis, and acupuncture. Feldenkrais, despite his refusal of surgery, succeeded in learning to walk again, and even resumed his judo. His months of careful minimal movements with disciplined self-observation enabled him to reawaken and refine young children's learning processes to move and function. In summary, he found that the key to healing was to become more "aware" of what one is doing.

He went on to regain full movement of his knee. Furthermore, he helped a friend and fellow scientist to similarly recover from severe, chronic back pain.

We now understand, especially from our personal trainer here in Duncan, Judy Lamontagne, the ability of our body to adapt and take "shortcuts" or "easy solutions." This occurs frequently in weight training, and Judy and her staff ensure that the desired maneuver is always consistent. This is especially critical in our walking and gait. When the body loses a muscle or group thereof, due to MS, it usually makes do or substitutes a movement to "replace" the other. Unfortunately, this often complicates our gait and sometimes reduces our strength, joint mobility, and mobility options. Then, when we recruit new nerve pathways, through our focus and effort, the muscle may recover, but our gait does not. In other words, the body still uses the "shortcut" it had adapted to and ignores the recovery of a normal gait. It is up to us to seek out a knowledgeable trainer, physiotherapist,

Feldenkrais-trained individual or a specialist like Meir Schneider to permit normal gait and walking again.

For anyone with MS who is still quite mobile, I suggest doing a modest amount of "training" in one form or another to keep it that way. Yoga, chi gong, and especially tai chi are also wonderful modalities. We started tai chi some months ago and firmly believe that if someone learns the series of movements and focuses on them for one to two hours a week, the results will be awesome. Tai chi is a set of moves that become almost reflex, after some 1,000 correct repetitions. This recruits and trains many of our "backup" and "dormant" spinal and brain pathways. Subsequently, if MS injures some of our original pathways, we will have these other tai chi–trained pathways ready and waiting.

CHAPTER SIXTEEN

Depression, Cognition, Brain Fog, and Suicide

The person afflicted with MS comes to personally understand the fragile ecosystem of the human brain. Fortunately, we have been able to learn some useful ideas and patterns that may help us regain and maintain hope.

Years of experience have shown that depression is more common with most any brain "injury" or illness. Other ones include not only stroke and brain trauma (e.g., head injury) but also degenerative diseases such as ALS, Parkinson's, and Alzheimer's.

Fifty percent of people diagnosed with MS will sustain a major depression sometime following diagnosis. Before the diagnosis, our risk is only 15%. Battles with depression can even appear prior to the diagnosis of MS. These episodes of depression can be treated with imipramine, our oldest (50-60 years) tricyclic antidepressant. Despite ongoing medication, I had one very bad time, four to five months after leaving work, when I got into a bottle of Scotch to "solve" my troubles. Fortunately, our son Brian put me to bed and removed the whiskey bottle. Depression and alcohol are a terrible mixture, as they can result in a downward spiral.

Fifty percent of people diagnosed with MS will sustain a major depression sometime following diagnosis.

The number one cause of death in people diagnosed with MS is suicide. Why? We have already lost three very close friends with MS to this "loss of hope" endpoint. One friend was a successful professional, divorced twice since his MS diagnosis, who wanted out of life before he got worse. He was pushing away his close relationships to distance himself from pity. As he moved toward despair and lost hope of recovery, he sought death as his exit, while he was still physically capable. A second friend had to leave work as MS had reduced her cognitive skills—gone was her ability to problem-solve. She was living evidence of how MS could severely limit the multitasking that modern life requires of us. We now know that most likely to commit suicide are the successful, determined individuals. When they decide to take a course of action, they invariably succeed.

Some 65% of people with MS have the "invisible" but very real disability of cognitive difficulties.

Excessive depression can lead to despair, and suicide can present itself as a solution. I had been very close to this state of despair. After more than a year of sliding downhill with my MS, the concept of suicide seemed a shortcut. We are now incredibly grateful that everyone hung in there and rallied. Once small steps of improvement occurred, the feelings of hope return.

Brain Fog

Some 65% of people with MS have the "invisible" but very real disability of cognitive difficulties. This "brain fog" is the relative inability to quickly solve a complex problem, or even prioritize well a set of simultaneous problems. It can show up as trouble remembering sequences, such as directions, and learning to adapt. Certainly, if depression exists on top of this, it seriously compounds the problem. The loss of concentration, associated with depression, can be minimized once the depression is treated. All of us need to work to optimize our day and minimize our stresses to reduce the risk of depression recurrence. Optimal MS recovery requires personal and peer support, in conjunction with vitamin D, light therapy, psychotherapy, and, when needed, antidepressant medication. The specter of suicide will always linger, and therefore must be a consideration in times of high stress from any cause.

Sunlight and Vitamin D

Solutions for depression increase as nutrition and health knowledge move forward. For example, reduced sunlight in fall, winter, and early spring can lead to Seasonal Affective Disorder (SAD), a depressed mood. Light therapy can help SAD. The light used provides full-spectrum illumination and is used 15-20 minutes daily. Light therapy can be a useful tool in beating back feelings of depression. A study done in Vancouver at the Women's Hospital revealed that this light therapy much reduced the incidence of postpartum depression. Other studies confirm the improvement in mood with light therapy. It is now understood that full-spectrum light, bright enough, or long enough daily, raises melatonin production. Melatonin is the precursor, or building block, of serotonin and other neurotransmitter substances in the brain.

A second, more recent discovery is that vitamin D deficiency can aggravate depression. Recent data shows that reduced absorption occurs in some of us and we may need more vitamin D. Studies also show that many people in Canada have low blood levels of vitamin D as well as low intake of vitamin D—containing foods. Further compounding the problem is the tendency for people to seek shade during the summer months, cover up exposed skin, and apply sunscreens. Certainly, the RDIs of 400 IU for adults under age 70 and 600 IU for those over age 70 are not adequate (see Chapter 5 on vitamin D).

Deeper Understanding of Grief and Hope

Counseling, grief work, and relationship enhancement can all help counter depression. First of all, we need to seek a Higher Power to forgive ourselves. Second, we have to learn to like ourselves for who we are, rather than rely on our work to define our self-worth. Often a full-steam-ahead, workaholic, type-A person uses work done or achievements to maintain self-esteem. Again, this returns to the mind, body, and spirit growth paradigm. Helpful books include those by Deepak Chopra, Michael Greenwoods, Bernie Siegel, and a host of others who all speak about this personal, yet very important journey. There is always life—but despair and depression can blind our hope.

We could all benefit from a recently published book *The Last Taboo: A Survival Guide to Mental Health Care in Canada,* by Scott Simmie and Julia Nunes. We like the book's candor as it discusses the frequency of mental disorders, diagnosis and solutions, drugs and alternatives, and suicide—the last taboo. We particularly appreciate the final chapter stressing the importance of all humans having "a home, a job, and a friend." No matter our illness or wellness, we are all complex and spiritual beings and not islands unto ourselves.

The Mental Health Association of Canada describes, *The Last Taboo* as "the best and most practical book ever written about mental illness and mental health in Canada" and states that it will "do more than any previous publication to break down the fear and stigma surrounding people with psychiatric disabilities and encourage them and their families to take control of their lives." We believe a similar "control of their lives" is equally important for people with MS and other illnesses. Simmie and Nunes point out that "recovery does not mean cure. . . . It is about living again, in a world beyond diagnosis. About regaining our rightful place in society."

Multiple Sclerosis, Diagnosis, Medical Management and Rehabilitation, edited by Jack S. Burk, MD, and Kenneth P. Johnson, MD, contains a chapter on "Cognitive and Emotional Disorders" by Nicholas G. LaRocca, PhD. LaRocca writes of memory lapses, mood swings, grief, and depression. Injury to the brain by MS leads to cognitive dysfunction. These can be further subdivided into such items as perseverance (refusal to give up; continued effort, especially under a handicap); deficits in executive functions such as planning, prioritizing, and sequencing complex tasks; reduced speed of information processing; reduced verbal fluency; and spatial difficulties such as three-dimensional or map-reading tasks.

LaRocca continues to say that although severe clinical depression may be associated with mild cognitive impairment, there is little or no relationship between depression and cognitive deficits in folks with MS. Memory, both verbal and visual, is the most common problem in MS. In addition, though short-term memory is usually spared, working memory (i.e., the brief processing of information and temporary storage) is impaired. He states that abstract reasoning and problem-solving are also often impaired. Attention and concentration may be problematic, especially if the topic is complex and sustained attention is needed. The above comments help describe our trouble with driving directions and difficulty following them.

In summary, LaRocca states that MS may be thought of as undermining the overall organization of brain processes. Some studies have found little or no relationship between cognitive deficits and physical neurological impairment or duration. "In contrast, many studies have found that patients with a progressive course are at greater risk for cognitive changes." Finally, cognitive changes may occur at any time during MS and happen in both mildly and severely disabled individuals. In fact, persons with severe physical disability may be completely free of cognitive changes.

CHAPTER SEVENTEEN

Our Five Senses and Beyond

As humans living in complex and busy environments, we are often overwhelmed with sensory input. Bombarded with an endless stream of commercials and complex input from the media and the world at large, our bodies try to cope, until something goes awry. Many chronic illnesses have chronic pain or other disabling symptoms. This chapter provides clarity on a number of sensory issues that can crop up in someone with multiple sclerosis. Much of the information can also apply to other chronic illnesses.

Vision

Nearly 80% of people with MS are first diagnosed because of changes in vision. Vision is one of the most important senses we possess for retaining our independence. Probable loss of part, or all, of our vision is a most frightening experience. Why does vision loss occur so frequently?

The eye or optic nerve is a part of the brain and spinal cord (central nervous system). As such, it too is susceptible to our errant white blood cells attacking, or chewing away on, the myelin—the protective covering insulating our nerves. When this occurs, the body responds to the free radicals and cytokines with inflammation, the body's healing solution. As noted, inflammation (as with a sprained ankle) means swelling, heat, redness, and pain (or loss of function). Swelling has a devastating effect on the optic nerve, because the optic nerve travels through a narrow aperture or hole in our bony skull. A small amount of swelling can tem-porarily reduce or minimize vision from that eye. Also, shooting pain may be a secondary symptom of this inflammation.

During this stage of acute inflammation in MS, corticosteroids are often used by physicians. Other options include regular emu oil capsules, regular or periodic boosts of glutathione enhancement (with a whey protein isolate as discussed in Chapter 4), and the boosting of omega-3 fatty acids from flax and/or fish oils. In addition, omega-3s enhance tear production—especially important for someone with Sjogren's Syndrome (dry eyes and dry mouth) or for people who wear contact lenses or who are considering corneal surgery.

Improved nutrition can also protect and enhance our vision as we age. A diet high in natural antioxidants is the foundation for eye health. Specific supplements providing omega-3 fatty acids, lutein (minimum 2g/day), and bonded or bioactive cysteine (see Chapter 4 on glutathione for details) are especially important. These supplements can slow down, or even reverse, early cataracts and reduce our risk of macular degeneration and other eye problems (e.g., glaucoma, which is likely an auto-immune disease).

In addition, success in one part of our brain and spinal cord (CNS) pro-vokes similar improved well-being in other areas of the CNS. We too often forget that all of our body is linked with blood circulation, nerves, lymph flow, and hormones. This is why improvement in one region, organ, or sys-tem usually transfers benefits to others. An obvious link to vision is hearing. We know that by raising glutathione in the inner ear, we can often improve our sense of hearing. Similarly, this same boost of GSH unfolds cataract crystals! As mentioned in Chapter 15, people with MS become very eye dependent. Now we can look after our vision better as well!

Finally, please refer to Chapter 2 on vitamins and minerals. Some carotenoids that are key in vision are beta-carotene, zeaxanthin, and lutein. Therefore, in your health journey, consider eating a variety of whole fruits and vegetables for high carotenoid intake. More than 600 carotenoids are found in nature, and we know that at least 50 of these are important nutritionally. For added protection, select multivitamin and multi-mineral plant-based supplements that contain these carotenoids.

Proprioception

Proprioception is another important sense to highlight. As noted, this refers to knowing where our body parts—arms, legs, and trunk—are relative to one another. Most of us with MS become hugely dependent on our eyes to compensate for loss of proprioception. Our neurologists examine us and use two tests for proprioception. One is the Romberg test, done standing with feet together and arms outstretched in front, palms up. We then close our eyes. Healthy individuals maintain their balance. Those with loss of proprioception lose their balance.

For more than six years, I tended to fall on my butt. After "retraining" or recruiting backup miniature motor nerve (gamma) pathways, I am now pretty stable, even with my eyes closed. The second of these tests involves reaching from finger to nose and the neurologist's hand, quickly and repeatedly. I was awful at this but am much better now. Similarly, my eye-hand coordination, which relies on vision and proprioception, is better. Once again, I can enjoy table tennis and swatting houseflies reasonably well! By the way, poor-quality proprioception also increases our risk of falls. This is an important factor post-stroke and in ALS, MS, and even Parkinson's disease. Both vitamin D supplementation and retraining nerve pathways will help to decrease falls.

Touch

Touch is a well-recognized sense as well. When my MS was at its worst, I needed to check the temperature of the shower water with my shoulder. Similarly, I cannot determine the coldness in my hands and feet until they actually turn white and start to hurt. Loss of light touch has progressed to covering my entire body. We are still looking for ways to remedy or "retrain" this challenge. This change in touch is also a part of chronic pain. Chronic pain folks are hypersensitive to touch (hyperalgesic), due to the ends of nerves being exquisitely over-responsive. This again speaks of irritable or hypersensitive nerves. Hence, clothing or simply a light breeze can trigger excruciating pain. Remember, topical emu oil, at the time of shingles, cold sores, or genital herpes may provide sufficient relief to prevent "wind up" of long-term pain—the sooner applied the better.

Hearing

Hearing is one of our earliest sensations. Good-quality hearing is developed long before vision becomes dominant. This might explain our acoustic expertise in water, a skill we share with our fellow mammals such as dolphins and whales. For decades, operating room personnel have been taught that hearing is often our last sense to disappear and our first to come back under anesthesia. Making positive comments about the person "asleep" makes for better healing, less pain, and quicker recovery than making negative ones. Unfortunately, negative comments and jokes about obesity are, in my anesthesiology experience, common.

Hearing is supplied by a "double" nerve—balance and auditory. The "balance component," or "semicircular canals," affects many of us with MS. I now look back on a day with the kids at an amusement park outside Calgary on a roller coaster ride. The ride went round and round, and up and down. I not only got nauseated and had wobbly knees, but this condition persisted for 12 hours. In retrospect, we believe this persistence and easy nausea, which increased in my 30s, was likely MS.

Many of us with MS believe that our problem with balance is also associated with our "balance nerve" or vestibular nerve from our semicircular or balance canals. Instead, it may also be related to our loss of proprioception (knowing where our limbs are in relation to our body). As noted, we become very eye or vision dependent when we begin to lose our balance. By the way, the health of our nerve cells in the inner ear can be helped by taking antioxidants, especially glutathione.

Hearing is not as frequently affected in MS as vestibular or semicircular canal balance. However, it is not uncommon during an MS attack to be hypersensitive to hearing, so that any sound jangles us. *Jangles* is not a medical term. What we mean is that certain sounds or even rhythms seem to acutely irritate folks with MS and can make us very uncomfortable with our surroundings. This, too, is a hypersensitivity, where the hearing mechanism is not blunted but is more irritable than normal. My newest toy to reduce unpleasant noise is a special pair of headphones with Acoustic Noise Canceling properties. They are superb on airplanes and even in the dentist's chair. They cancel out much of the unpleasant sound and yet they still permit conversation. These are a great asset if traveling in noisy surroundings, as they secondarily reduce fatigue.

We have a good friend, Gill, who has major hearing problems with MS. She is a nurse and is nearly deaf due to MS injury to both inner ears (the acoustic collecting nerve within the brain). In fact, this must be exceedingly rare, for upon review by an experienced MS neurologist, she was referred, expeditiously, to an Ear, Nose and Throat (ENT) specialist. This ENT specialist examined her, repeated her MRI, and reassured her it was definitely due to her MS. The most striking feature of this is that the MS neurologist had given Gill the same referral, with the same ENT surgeon, with the same outcome, two to three years earlier!

Music is an underused option for recovery that we can try. We know that different types of music are pleasant or unpleasant to us individually. In addition, music by Mozart has been shown to calm the brain (even to an alpha rhythm), like meditation, to enhance learning. When my hearing is hypersensitive or "jangled," it is usually classical music that works best. This can even include the different tonic sounds of Asia or India. We believe learning music, via playing tuba, tenor saxophone, or voice, will help the brain recruit new pathways. My newest goal in music is to play the Irish harp, and to sing with it too!

Speech

Voice is probably the most challenging of all our senses, as our personal breathing, vocal cord position, emotion, and mouth muscles are all involved in speech. When my brother Stewart, a singer and musician, died in 1994, my grief at my loss made it nearly impossible for me to sing for almost a year. We believe music can be a very useful tool to help enhance our mind-body-spirit connection. In addition, optimal breathing can help not just our singing voice, but can also significantly help improve our speech in MS in the long term. Working with music's pitch and tone stimulates hearing. This, in turn, will help our speech. Choir lessons will much improve our breathing patterns to protect our speaking abilities. Yoga is quite helpful as well.

Taste

Taste is another of our five senses. In fact, we have only four major taste buds (sweet, sour, bitter, and salty) and five minor ones. This relative lack of taste buds further reminds us of the importance of planning a well-balanced diet with supplements. We cannot rely solely on taste to ensure that we meet our nutrient needs. We are programmed, by evolution, to enjoy fat and sweet. However, a diet of doughnuts and french fries does not provide us with all the nutrients for health. Sometimes, too, we crave foods. Pica is the extreme in craving; people with pica have been known to eat clay or to chew relentlessly on ice cubes. It is thought that pica might be the body's response to a nutrient deficiency. For example, the ice craving usually declines with iron supplementation. In contrast to our limited taste buds, dogs and horses have some 200 taste buds, and cows and emus are believed to have 500! Hence, unlike animals, humans cannot instinctively search out needed nutrients important to survival. We need to plan to eat a variety of foods every day. Thus, wisdom and nutrition education can be very helpful so that we have the right balance of foods and supplements to optimize our health and recovery from MS or other chronic diseases.

Taste is essential for our enjoyment of food. Anything interfering with our sense of smell can result in a diminished sense of taste. Thus, taste and smell are closely linked. In addition, many drugs can interfere with our ability to taste and smell foods. Some drugs can alter how foods taste. Other drugs may decrease saliva and cause a loss of taste sensation. So, be aware of any changes in taste or smell when you take new medications and report them to your doctor. People who have changes in taste or smell often eat less. A reduced food intake might cause inadequate intake of important nutrients.

Smell

Even though smell is perhaps our oldest and longest established sense, we rarely consider it in regular Western medicine. A wide spectrum of smelling abilities exists among people—some are super sniffers, some average sniffers, and others minimal sniffers. When I smell certain irritating or pungent, unpleasant smells, I often make tracks to avoid them. Whenever I ignore this sensation I might pay dearly for it with a migraine headache. The upside of our sense of smell is that there are also pleasant smells. Aromatherapy is commonly practiced in Europe and on the west coast of North America, and is spreading to all parts of the globe. I now accept that this is more than just an incredible perfume or "scent of a woman," but, in fact, it has some safe, simple advantages for those of us with MS.

Aromatherapy is an ancient form of healing using pure essential oils extracted from flowers, leaves, petals, blossoms, bark, trees, roots, twigs, seeds, berries, resins, and rinds. The oils are very powerful and effective, and are what gives the plants their fragrance. These highly volatile oils are sensitive to heat and light, contain hormones and vitamins, are soluble in alcohol and oil, and are not water soluble.

Acting on the central nervous system, essential oils stimulate the body's natural ability to heal itself, balance the body, and to rejuvenate and calm mind, body, and spirit.

Acting on the central nervous system, essential oils stimulate the body's natural ability to heal itself, balance the body, and to rejuvenate and calm mind, body, and spirit. These essential oils can be administered through massage, in baths or showers, and as room fragrances.

Some randomized controlled trials have suggested that the oils of certain flowers (such as lavender) may have antidepressant and anti-anxiety properties. Aromatherapy is an effective complementary therapy for helping to manage chronic pain. "Essential oils are like a team of good friends, all helping out in the best way they can when their particular attributes are needed."[1] "In ancient Greece aromatic oils were often employed for their sleep inducing, antidepressant, or aphrodisiac properties, and it was recognized that certain odours could improve mental alertness and aid concentration."[2]

Methods of Application

METHOD OF APPLICATION	AMOUNT OF ESSENTIAL OIL	AMOUNT OF CARRIER OIL OR WATER
Massage (full body)	10-15 drops	25 ml/1 oz. oil
Massage (localized area)	15-20 drops	10 ml carrier oil
Bath	6-10 drops	1 tsp carrier oil in full tub of water
Inhalation (steam)	3-5 drops	Bowl of boiled water
Inhalation (tissue)	2-3 drops	n/a
Diffuser	6-8 drops	Water as required
Room Sprayer	10-15 drops	100 ml water
Compress	4-6 drops	Bowl of water

[1] Valerie Ann Worwood, *The Fragrant Pharmacy*, (New York: Bantam Books, 1993), 98.
[2] Robert Tisserand, *Aromatherapy for Everyone* (London: Arkana, 1990).

If you are interested in learning more about aromatherapy, essential oil applications, and which oils to use, do your research and/or consult an aromatherapist before beginning your adventure with essential oils.

NOTE: It is important to purchase 100% pure essential oils from a reputable supplier.

Before leaving aromatherapy, I would like to include one more plant: cistus ladaniferus. French aromatherapy experts particularly recommend this essential oil for reducing the fatigue of MS. I am trying this out personally. Watch our website, www.drbillcode.com, for further updates.

Psycho-Aromatherapy

On Friday, 10 September 2004, at the British Psychological Society's Division of Health Psychology Annual Conference in Edinburgh, new research by psychologists revealed the positive effects of aromatherapy on the quality of life for multiple clerosis (MS) sufferers. These researchers, at the University of Teeside, in Middlesbrough, England, found MS patients, in spite of experiencing the same symptoms, felt more vitality, happiness, and peace during aromatherapy treatment, and less depression, fatigue, and anxiety. The authors say that the mechanism by which improvements in quality of life occurred is unknown, but that there is "growing evidence for the effectiveness of aromatherapy on chronic illness." This finding offers some hope that while a cure is sought for chronic illness, Health Psychology could help people to live with its effects in the long term.[1]

[1] The British Psychological Society (BPS), Essential Hope for Multiple Sclerosis, Division of Health Psychology, BPS Press Office, 17 September 2004; Ref. PR645

	Aphrodisiac
Essential Oils	Clary Sage Patchouli Jasmine Ylang Ylang
Type of Problems Relieved	Emotional Coldness, Shyness, Impotence, Frigidity
Neurochemical Secreted	ENDORPHINS
Part of Brain Triggered by Essential Oil	PITUITARY

Regulating	Euphoric	Memory/ Mental Stimulant	Sedative	Invigorating
Bergamot Geranium Frankincense Rosewood	Clary Sage Grapefruit Jasmine Rose Otto	Black Pepper Peppermint Lemon Rosemary	Chamomile Lavender Marjoram Orange Blossom	Cardamom Clary Sage Lemongrass Patchouli
Anxiety with Depression, Mood Swings, Menstrual or Menopausal Imbalance	Depression, Moodiness, Lack of Confidence	Mental Fatigue, Difficulty in Concentrating, Poor Memory	Anxiety, Stress, Hypertension, Insomnia, Anger, Irritability	Boredom, Lethargy, Immune Deficiency
VARIOUS	ENKEPHALINS	VARIOUS	SEROTONIN	NOR-ADRENALINE
HYPO-THALAMUS	THALAMUS	AMYGDALA & HIPPO-CAMPUS	RAPHE NUCLEUS	LOCUS CERULEUS

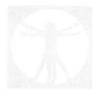

Where We Are Now and Where We Are Going

Both Denise and I indeed feel fortunate that we shared a great deal of knowledge and wisdom before the onset of my multiple sclerosis. Our marriage of 31-plus years has been enlightened and fueled by a master's degree in Nutrition on one side and extensive work in brain and stroke research, pharmacology, and physiology on the other. This synergy, combined with the much-improved communication in our world today, has made this book possible and we hope you find it worthwhile for you or someone you care about who may be on a personal journey with chronic pain, multiple sclerosis, or some other chronic illness. Our goal is to make this book a source of practical and usable health information, supplemented by updates at our web site, www.drbillcode.com.

We find ourselves tremendously blessed at this point in our lives. Our children, Warren, Brian, and Laura, are now in their 20s and have each completed college. Warren is on his way to achieving a PhD in math and enjoys teaching at the college level. Brian, a computer engineer, just decided to leave the corporate world to launch his own consulting firm and help us with our growing health wisdom business. Laura, a graduate in Agriculture with an Animal Science specialty, has just accepted a job with the Ministry of Agriculture in British Columbia. She will be working as a Youth and Community Development Specialist and will be supporting the 4H program. They remain very close as siblings and have grown into strong, compassionate, and caring adults who have much to contribute to making this a better world.

At this time, life is indeed full. We have attended many seminars in the past two years to improve our business skills, enhance our health knowledge, and become better educators. We love learning and we love sharing our knowledge! Thus, we offer health seminars and individual counseling to continue spreading information and hope. Each week we receive emails and phone calls from people who are looking for answers to their health problems. We also continue to actively farm emus and market emu oil and other health products under the Songlines Health Products label.

Life is fun, challenging, and full of family, friends, and the wonderful people we meet as we travel. Our passion for what we do often leads to long hours and road trips away from home but we know we are making a difference in so many lives. This keeps us enlivened and eager to move forward. No one is sure what the future will bring, but we anticipate wonderful things. We are upgrading our website to serve the public better and are also planning to host teleconferences and web seminars so that we can reach more people. A regular newsletter is also in the works. And who knows … another book?

We hope we have provided you with all of the inspiration, information, and tools you'll need to get on the road to recovery and optimal health. Work with your healthcare practitioners—physicians, nurse practitioners, naturopaths or otherwise—but, remember, make them your coaches, not dictators.

Just consider the possibility that what you learn, reflect on, or discuss with others can have a major value on your personal journey to health. We realize this may be scary or challenge your beliefs, but we are here to guide your growth. To help you with this, both Denise and I are now providing teleseminars. Occasionally, the teleseminars feature Alesandra Rain and the advice for drug taper from Point of Return. Future teleseminars will be held in collaboration with other health experts. By the time you read this book, we will have progressed to coaching, workshops, and, ultimately, a healing spa opportunity. Benefits to you will include:

1. A return to self-confidence and decision-making that empowers you.

2. You and your partner will become your own best caregiver.

3. Reduced pain for you, at both a physical and emotional level.

4. A healthy nutrition and lifestyle change you enjoy and that agrees with you personally.

5. A road map that is practical and achievable in your journey to health.

I have joined the Associate Fellowship Training Program in Integrative Medicine at the University of Arizona. It is led by Executive Director Dr. Victoria Maize, MD, and originator, Dr. Andrew Weil, MD. Wisdom gained here will be shared with not only health care professionals and students, but also the concerned and searching person—you, on your life journey.

Our support and coaching programs will allow gradual progression, at your chosen speed, and your pocketbook. The variety will include a newsletter (online or mail), telephone consultation, Frequently Asked Questions seminars over the web, live speaking contact, and hands-on workshops, and even a healing spa. You can determine what you need or want, at your pace. Your journey is in your own hands, and even small steps can and will make a difference.

We salute your progress to date and sincerely appreciate your effort in reading our book. Please visit our website www.drbillcode.com or call 1-888-746-1593.

For the ultimate short summary you will note Dr. Bill's Top 10 Supplement Choices for Reversing Aging, Reducing Pain, and Improving Energy and Brain Function, found on page 107. You can send for a copy, with a self-addressed, stamped envelope, or get it online at www.drbillcode.com (see *Appendix A & B*).

Contact Us

Dr. Bill Code, MD
Denise Code, MSc, RD
Box 877
Duncan, B.C. V9L 3Y2
Canada

drbill@drbillcode.com
denise@drbillcode.com

www.winningthepaingame.com
www.drbillcode.com
www.askdrbillcode.com

International: 1-250-746-7080
In the USA and Canada: 1-888-746-1593
Fax: 1-250-746-4803

What People Are Saying

Peaks and Valleys of My Journey
By Jeannette Hughes

At 32 years of age, with five children under 10, I was diagnosed with multiple sclerosis. (I had my first attack eight years earlier, in 1963, but the small prairie hospital where I was treated failed to recognize the MS symptoms.) I have managed to keep myself going and accomplish a great deal despite all odds.

In 2004, I am a widow, working usually 14- to 16-hour days as a Sidney town councilor, and also an extremely active participant in many other aspects of the community. Although I have never said my life as a person with MS has been easy—far from it—I usually dwell on the peaks rather than the valleys.

During the first 10 years after I received the fateful news of my chronic illness, I experienced a significant attack requiring hospitalization every year. Severe loss of vision several times, numbness to the point that I had no feeling in my body from my neck down, and then a severe drug reaction disabled me further. Following one attack, I could not even write my name for six months and could not drive for 48 months although I later got behind an automobile wheel again for several years and, more recently, became so proficient on a scooter that I produced a video and wrote a pamphlet on scooter safety). I also wrestled with severe depression, partly because I had little moral support from a family who had trouble accepting my health situation. Rest, antidepressants and steroids were not the answer.

Trying to find answers for myself during this "dark decade," I met several people with MS and started the first MS support group in the area of

Vancouver Island where I then lived—which still is going strong after 30 years. Through the group, I found the courage to get back on my feet after every major attack, survive five teenagers, go to university, change my career from nursing to research and writing for the provincial Ministry of Health, divorce and live on my own for three years. I subsequently co-authored one book and authored another, prepared various pamphlets and guides, and wrote published articles about self-motivation and strategies for coping with adversity. In addition, I remarried, travelled and changed careers again . . . and even did some television production and became something of an expert in universal design.

The list of alternative therapies I have tried is so long I will mention only a few: pool therapy (swimming and water exercise), hot tub exercise, working with a trainer at the Body Barn Gym in Sidney (much more fun than a PT at the MS clinic), journal-writing, meditation (TM), visualization, dance therapy and laser acupuncture (which cured seven years of severe back pain). As well, I have experimented with various supplements.

Part of my survival strategies have been, resisting medical suggestions to go on drug trials, take pain killers, "just rest," use a back brace, and take steroids and numerous other drugs. Keeping an open positive mind and gaining control over my MS has allowed me to live an active fulfilled life. Of the supplements I have tried, the most dramatic results have been from the whey protein isolate (see Chapter 4).

More than 15 years ago, while cutting back my juniper bushes, my legs became severely scratched and bleeding, as I had no feeling in them. After six months on a particular whey protein isolate providing bioactive cysteine, one day an ant ran up my leg and I felt every tiny footprint. I realized that after all those years I was regaining feeling in my legs. The foregoing is just a glimpse of my life, which has been enhanced in the past few years through the caring and constructive influence of Dr. William Code. It is a privilege to have this opportunity to thank him in print.

— Jeannette

Dear William Code,

We met at a Rotary meeting in Duncan last summer. I was visiting rotarian from Denmark. You where kind to give me a copy of your book about MS, and I just want to let you know, that your book already has helped some people in Denmark.

In August last year one of my colleagues wife had the diagnosis MS. I lent her your book, and she found hope in it. She is age 39 and the mother of 3 children. She is now back in her job and living a normal life.

Last week the wife of a friend of mine had the same diagnosis. She is age 42. I, am sending her your book today confident that it will help her also.

I just wanted to let you know.

Yours in Rotary

— Jurgen Burk

I have had CFS/ME (Chronic Fatigue Syndrome/Myalgic Encephalomyelitis) for 8 years. During this time I have tried numerous supplements and remedies to no avail. About 4 years ago Dr. Code introduced me to a specialized whey protein powder. Wow, what a difference! I will not go a day without it. My energy levels have improved and overall I have experienced a better sense of well being. It also has helped with my IBS (Irritable Bowel Syndrome). I still need to rest during the day, but without this specialized whey protein, I would definitely be spending more time in bed. This is a great product!

— Earl Kamer

Bill,

Great to see you today, thank you for the emu oil pills and the CD, also the stuff that doesn't taste so well. Had some—you're right!!

Who's in Control of Your Multiple Sclerosis?: a wonderful book for someone to learn all about MS and to not be scared of it. It has helped me a great deal. It is an illness that can be controlled. Bill is living proof.

Keep in touch,

All the best

(Name withheld due to confidentiality)

Dear Bill and Denise,

Good morning from M&M in sunny Sooke.

Great to see you yesterday and a very special thank you for your new book (Who's in Control of Your Multiple Sclerosis)*; it is very much appreciated. Your lectures are an inspiration to all of us.*

I admire your determination to climb the MS ladder versus slipping down the ladder. I too have tried to do the same, mostly through diet. After I study your new book in detail, I would like to discuss what you are doing that may also be of help to me. Many thanks again.

Sincerely,

— Marion Vanderwood

Dear Bill and Denise,

I have read your books but when I finished the last book you gave me, when we were at Edgar and Ruby's, I was so overwhelmed by your story I cannot help but write to you. Your thoughts, your pain, the frustration, and how your have worked your way to what you are today is truly an amazing victory.

Years ago when I first heard you had MS you were in my thoughts very often. I prayed that you might be able to help carry on and use your talents.

Thank God, that has happened with much effort on your part, you didn't give up and I marvel how energetic you are.

I pray for your future years that you can keep on doing what you are doing now.

Bill and Denise, you will always be in my thoughts and prayers!

Sincerely

With love

— Tina Harder

Suggested Reading, Resources, and Supplies

Books

Benson, Herbert. *The Relaxation Response.* New York: Harper Torch, 1976.

Code, William E., and Claudia Tiefisher. *Youth Renewed.* Calgary, Alberta, Canada: Chameleon Publishing, 2000.

Code, William E., and Denise Code. *Who's in Control of your Multiple Sclerosis?* Montreal, Canada: AGMV-Marquis Imprimeur, Inc, 2005.

Davis, Brenda, and Tom Barnard. *Defeating Diabetes.* United States: Healthy Living Publications, 2003.

Graci, Sam. *The Food Connection.* Toronto, Canada: Macmillan Canada, 2001.

Graci, Sam. *The Path to Phenomenal Health.* Canada: John Wiley & Sons, 2005.

Kabat-Zinn, Jon. *Wherever You Go, There You Are: Mindfulness Meditation in Everyday Life.* New York: Hyperion, 1995.

King, Brad J. *Awaken Your Metabolism.* Ontario, Canada: Health Venture Publications, 2005.

Nestle, Marion. *What to Eat.* New York: North Point Press, 2006.

Rain, Alesandra, Andrea Crocker, and Dr. Bill Code. *Point of Return: Your Personal Guide to Taper Off Anti-Anxiety & Anti-Depressant Drugs.* Malibu, CA: Label Me Sane, Inc., 2006.

Servan-Schreiber, David. *The Instinct to Heal.* Rodale Inc., 2004.

Weil, Andrew. *8 Weeks to Optimum Health: A Proven Program for Taking Full Advantage of Your Body's Natural Healing Power.* New York: Ballantine, 2006.

Weil, Andrew. *Eating Well for Optimum Health: The Essential Guide to Bringing Health and Pleasure Back to Eating.* New York: Harper Collins, 2001.

Weil, Andrew. *Spontaneous Healing: How to Discover and Enhance your Body's Natural Ability to Maintain and Heal Itself.* New York: Ballantine, 2000.

Williams, Montel, with Lawrence Grobel. *Climbing Higher.* New American Library, 2004.

Williams, Montel, and Wini Linquvic. *Body Change.* Mountain Movers Press, 2001.

Newsletter

Dr. Bill Code's Health Wisdom
5816 Menzies Road
Duncan, B.C. V9L 6J9

www.drbillcode.com
drbill@drbillcode.com
www.askdrbillcode.com

1-888-746-1593
1-250-746-7080

Websites

1. www.winningthepaingame.com
2. www.drbillcode.com
3. www.pointofreturn.com
4. www.integrativemedicine.arizona.edu
5. www.ninds.nih.gov/disorders/chronic_pain/chronic_pain
6. www.msbiketours.com
7. www.MarkVictorHansen.com

The "Winning" & Health Recovery Series

No Matter Where You Start,
Dr. Bill Code Can Help You on Your Health Journey

Books

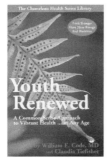

Youth Renewed: A common sense approach to health at any age

The common sense approach in this book is like a breath of fresh air in the mountain of health information available today.

ISBN   978-0-9687668-0-4

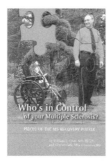

Who's in Control of Your Multiple Sclerosis? Pieces of the MS Recovery Puzzle

An essential guide to hope and recovery. This book's emphasis is on safe, effective, natural solutions based on sound scientific evidence. Learn how you can control your MS so that MS does not control you.

ISBN   978-0-9787463-6-0

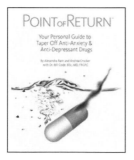

Point of Return; Your Personal Guide To Taper Off Anti-Anxiety & Anti-Depressant Drugs

ISBN   978-0-9778040-1-6

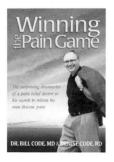

Winning the Pain Game: The Surprising Discoveries Of A Pain Relief Doctor In His Search To Relieve His Own Chronic Pain

ISBN   978-0-9787463-0-8

Digital Books
(Downloadable electronic books)

Who's In Control of Your MS?
  Pieces of the MS Recovery Puzzle
    ISBN 978-0-9787463-1-5

Winning the Pain Game
    ISBN 978-0-9787463-2-2

Books on Audio CDs or MP3

Who's in Control of Your MS?
  Pieces of the MS Recovery Puzzle
        Audio CD ISBN   978-0-9787463-3-9
        MP3 ISBN   978-0-9787463-7-7

Winning the Pain Game
        Audio CD ISBN   978-0-9787463-4-6
        MP3 ISBN   978-0-9787463-8-4

Home Study Program

Winning the Pain Game Home Study Course

In this home study audio program packed with how-to tips, Dr. Bill will personalize your pain recovery journey. You will be coached by Dr. Bill as though he is with you in your home, car, or office. Each step of the journey, be it food changes, supplements, or education on label and product decisions, will contribute to your pain reduction

- 10 extraordinary audio sessions (CD's and MP3 versions)

- Exclusive Bonus session on Sleep

- Accompanying workbooks on CD Rom

Best of all, with Winning the Pain Game Home Study Course, you will have Dr. Bill as your personal one on one, pain reduction coach. Through these audio sessions he'll be available to you whenever you need him, so you'll never forget your focus or lose momentum. You can check in anytime you want principle explained, a shot of energy, or a fresh dose of inspiration. And you can listen anywhere – while commuting, traveling – or even walking or exercising.

Also included in the Winning the Pain Game Home Study Course is a signed copy of "Winning the Pain Game".

ISBN 978-0-9787463-5-3

Audio CDs
60 Minutes

- Multiple Sclerosis and Chronic Pain
- Improving Brain Function and Whey Protein Isolate Implications
- Emu Oil

- Anti-anxiety Medication Taper (Benzodiazepines)
- Multiple Sclerosis & Personal Supplement Choices
- Are You On An Antidepressant? What Is Your Biggest Concern Taking It? with Guest Speaker Alesandra Rain
- Sleep

**To order any of the above resources,
visit www.WinningThePainGame.com
or www.DrBillCode.com**

Take your health to the next level...

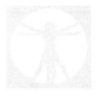

Health Supplements

We recommend and use a variety of sources. These are best found at the website and phone numbers below:

www.songlineshealthproducts.com
Phone: 1-888-784-2244
International: 1-250-746-7080
Fax: 1-250-746-4803

- Emu Oil Products:

  CalEmu: Marine calcium, magnesium, trace minerals and collagen, for joint health

  Emu Oil Gel Caps: anti-inflammatory, helps fatigue, thicken scalp hair

  Emu-Omega-3: Emu Oil and Omega-3 blend, unique on the market

  Joint Comfort: for muscle spasm and joint pain, cream base

  Natural Body Rub/Emu Oil: pure emu oil, nothing added, the most hypoallergenic

  Natural Face Care: creamy and luxurious; ideal for pre-wrinkles and wrinkles

  Skin Repair: dry hands, feet, elbows, acne, rosacea, post shaving

  Warm Body Rub: for muscle and joint pain, emu oil base

  Lip Balm: all natural lip balm contains emu oil and beeswax to help dry, chapped lips, cold sores or canker sores.

- Whey Protein Isolate, PROTECT. Note: Dr. Bill and Denise Code helped formulate PROTECT, especially for brain recovery and tapering off of tranquilizers and antidepressant drugs as guided by your physician.
- CALM
- Digestive Enzymes
- Infrared Saunas
- Omega-3 Oils, Flax, and MOOD
- Prebiotics and Probiotics
- Tart Montmorency Cherry Extract
- Vitamin/Mineral Supplements

www.immunotec.com/essentialfood
1-604-740-8275

For: Immunocal (whey protein isolate)
     Immunocal Platinum (whey protein isolate)
     Magistral (saw palmetto)
     Xtra Sharp (herbal energy tonic)
     PNT200 (milk peptide for stress management)
     Milk Calcium
     Fruit and Vegetable Capsules

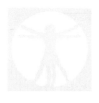

Glossary

absorb – (nutrition) to draw nutrients from the gastrointestinal tract into the bloodstream.

acquired immune deficiency syndrome (AIDS) – a deficiency in the immune system due to infection by the human immunodeficiency virus (HIV).

ADHD – Attention Deficit Hyperactivity Disorder: a condition characterized by inability to concentrate, focus, or sit still. Often medicated with *Ritalin*. Has been linked to a deficiency in omega-3 fatty acids.

aerobic exercise – any physical activity that makes the heart and lungs work harder to meet the muscles' need for oxygen.

albumin – a major protein found in blood serum.

allergy – an inappropriate immune response to a non-pathogen.

alveoli – tiny air sacs of the lungs, where carbon dioxide leaves the blood and oxygen is taken on by the blood.

Alzheimer's – a degenerative disorder caused by prolonged free radicals.

amino acids – organic chemical compounds from which all proteins are made.

anaerobic exercise – any physical activity in which oxygen is used by the muscles faster than it can be supplied by the bloodstream.

anaphylaxis – a sudden and rapid swelling of the body, especially breathing and airway. Usually an allergic response.

anemia – low hemoglobin (red blood cell) count.

anesthesiologist – a doctor of medicine graduate who studies five years to specialize in caring for people during surgery, intensive care, and pain management (e.g., labour, surgical, and trauma pain).

anthocyanins – any of several water-soluble nitrogenous pigments that contribute to the red, blue, or violet colors in some plants (e.g., cherries, grapes, plums). Powerful antioxidants.

antigen – a substance foreign to the body that triggers an immune response.

antigen response – the immune system's response to an antigen.

anti-inflammatory – a drug or compound that reduces the symptoms of inflammation.

antioxidant – a substance that neutralizes destructive free radicals or prevents oxidation; some are manufactured by the body, others are derived from foods.

arthritis – inflammation of joints characterized by pain, swelling, and stiffness, sometimes leading to deformation of the joint.

asthma – recurrent bouts of breathlessness of varying severity due to constriction of the small airways.

atherosclerotic plaque – a fatty or waxy substance that builds up in arteries leading to arteriosclerosis (hardening of the arteries).

auto-immune disease – a dysfunctional immune response to healthy processes; a disorder caused by inappropriate immune response to one's own tissue.

auto-immune disorder – one of a large group of diseases marked by a change of the immune system of the body. The body's defense system is turned against the body itself, causing chronic and often deadly diseases; many of these disorders have now been linked to allergies.

B. bifidus – a beneficial bacteria that lives in the gut.

bad fats (damaging) – *trans* (hydrogenated or partially hydrogenated) dietary fats, especially when consumed in excess.

B-cell lymphocyte – lymphocytes that manufacture antibodies.

beta-carotene – a precursor of vitamin A, found in carrots, tomatoes, etc., and converted in the body to vitamin A.

bioactivity – the initiation of specific metabolic activity by a nutrient or other compound.

bioavailability – the amount of a biological substance available for a bodily process.

biochemical – chemical compounds produced by or interacting with the body.

blood sugar – the amount of glucose in the blood.

cancer – a group of diseases characterized by unrestricted growth of cells in a tissue or specific organ.

candida – thrush or moniliasis; a fungal infection of the vagina or other areas of mucous membrane or moist skin.

carcinogen – a cancer-causing agent.

carotenoid – yellow or red pigments such as carotenes found widely in plants and animals.

carrier oils – used in aromatherapy, carrier oils are generally cold-pressed vegetable oils. Some examples are sweet almond, apricot kernel, grapeseed, avocado, peanut, olive, pecan, macadamia nut, sesame, evening primrose, and walnut.

casein – a milk protein; one of the products in milk.

cataract – the loss of transparency of the lens of the eye due to changes in the delicate protein fibers within the lens.

cell – the basic structural element of the body; trillions in number and highly differentiated in function.

cerebro-spinal fluid – a clear, watery liquid that surrounds and infuses the brain and the central canal of the spinal cord.

chelation – the attachment of toxins present in the body to organic compounds, allowing the toxins' excretion and resulting in diminished toxicity.

chelators – organic compounds that attract and stick to metal molecules.

cholesterol – an important fatty constituent of body cells; a player in the formation of hormones and the transport of fats to various parts of the body; HDL (good) cholesterol protects against arterial disease; LDL (bad) cholesterol promotes arterial disease.

chronic – of long duration; with diminished likelihood of cure.

chronic inflammatory change – persistent inflammation and its biochemical changes.

chronic inflammatory disease – persistent disease characterized by inflammation, such as rheumatoid arthritis.

cis fatty acid – a fatty acid configuration where the hydrogen atoms and the carbon atoms involved in the double bond are on the same side of the molecule, causing the molecule to bend or kink.

cold pressed – oils extracted from seeds or nuts without the use of hexane, and done at low temperatures.

colitis – general inflammation of the bowel.

collagen – the main protein substance of the body; responsible for the form and shape of most tissues (except bone and cartilage).

colon – the major part of the large intestine.

comedogenic (non-comedogenic) – acne-causing (non-acne causing).

complementary medicine – the combined application of conventional and alternative health practices.

complex carbohydrate – sugar molecules strung together to form longer, more complex chains. Complex carbohydrates include starch and fiber.

constipation – infrequent and difficult passing of hard feces.

cosmeceutical – a cross between a "cosmetic" and a "pharmaceutical"; a cosmetic product that is expected to have some therapeutic or active beneficial component(s).

cysteine – a sulfur-containing amino acid; the scarcest of the three constituents of GSH.

cystic fibrosis – mucoviscidosis; an inherited, congenital disease characterized by chronic lung infection and poor absorption of nutrients.

degenerative disease – physical and/or chemical changes in cells, tissues, or organs leading to progressive impairment of both structure and function.

delta-5-desaturase – an enzyme in the human body that converts components of fatty acids to "bad" eicosanoids. This enzyme is not present in the skin.

dementia – a general decline of mental functioning.

depression − feelings of sadness, hopelessness, pessimism, loss of interest in life, and diminished emotional well-being.

dermatitis − any mild or moderate inflammation of the skin causing rash and/or itchiness.

dermis − the thick layer of living tissue below the epidermis (skin).

desensitize − slowly and gradually reduce response (e.g., allergy to bee stings; fear of heights).

detoxifier − any substance that neutralizes toxins, pollutants, and carcinogens.

diarrhea − increased fluidity and frequency of bowel movements; a symptom of underlying disease.

disease − an unhealthy condition of the body or mind; illness, sickness.

dis-ease − an alternative medical practitioner's term for a state of the body that can be termed to be in *"dis"*-ease.

distress − stress beyond the body's ability to respond favorably.

diverticuli − tiny pouch-like sacs that develop in the colon, becoming inflamed when matter becomes lodged in them.

dopamine − a neurotransmitter found in the brain.

duodenum − first part of the small intestine, after the stomach.

dysfunction − abnormal activity; inability to function.

eclampsia − a rare, very serious condition of late pregnancy causing seizures and coma.

eczema − inflammation of the skin.

eicosanoids − hormone-like substances that regulate blood pressure, clotting, immune response, inflammation response, and other body functions; formed from omega-6 and omega-3 fatty acids.

emollient − a substance that softens tissues, especially the skin and mucous membranes.

emulsify − to mix a liquid into another liquid, making a suspension that has globules of fat.

emulsion − a mix of two liquids, made so that small droplets are formed, as oil and water.

emu oil – contains omega-3 and omega-6 essential fatty acids along with an anti-inflammatory pigment, probably a carotenoid. Can be ingested and/or used topically.

endogenous antioxidants – antioxidants produced within the body.

endorphins – the body's own natural painkillers.

enzyme – any protein that promotes or regulates a specific chemical reaction in the body.

Epstein-Barr virus – a DNA herpes virus that causes infectious mononucleosis.

essential amino acids – amino acids that must be obtained from dietary sources and cannot be manufactured by the body; arginine, histidine, isoleucine, leucine, lysine, methionine, phenylalanine, threonine, tryptophan, and valine.

essential fatty acids (EFAs) – several varieties of fatty acids that must be eaten because the body cannot manufacture them. Essential to brain function, manufacture of enzymes, and the integrity of the cell wall.

fat – nutrient providing the body with its most concentrated form of energy; a solid or liquid oil of vegetable or animal origin.

fiber – the indigestible portion of the diet consisting of various plant cell-wall materials, which passes through the body largely unchanged.

fiber foods – foods containing indigestible plant material that holds water and adds bulk to the feces, aiding normal bowel function.

fibroblasts – cells producing collagen fibers in connective tissue of the body.

flavonoids – a variety of crystalline compounds found in plants; some are powerful antioxidants.

flu (influenza) – contagious virus infection causing fever, severe aching, weakness, and coughing.

free radical – oxyradical; a highly reactive molecule with one or more unpaired electrons; free radical destruction is implicated in a wide variety of diseases.

GABA – gamma-aminobutyric acid; a neurotransmitter.

gingivitis – inflammation or infection of the gums accompanied by any combination of pain, swelling, and bleeding.

glaucoma – optic nerve fiber destruction and gradual loss of vision caused by increased fluid pressure within the eye.

glucagon – a polypeptide hormone formed in the pancreas, which aids the breakdown of glycogen to glucose in the liver.

glucose – a simple sugar containing six carbon atoms, which is an important energy source.

glutamine – a crystalline amino acid found in plant and animal protein.

glutathione (GSH) – a crystalline, water-soluble tripeptide composed of glutamic acid (glutamate), cysteine, and glycine.

glutathione peroxidase (GSH peroxidase) – an enzyme of glutathione critical as an antioxidant, especially against lipid peroxidation.

glycine – an amino acid and neurotransmitter.

glycogen – a polysaccharide serving as a store of carbohydrates, and yielding glucose on hydrolysis.

glycoproteins – any of a group of compounds consisting of a protein combined with a carbohydrate.

granulocyte – a type of white blood cell.

gut – the stomach and intestines.

hair follicles – small pits in the epidermis that grow individual hairs.

half-life – period required by the body to eliminate or metabolize a substance to 50% levels.

hexane – a chemical used to extract oil from seeds and nuts.

HDL cholesterol – high density lipoprotein; a component of blood that carries cholesterol but protects against arteriosclerosis; also known as "good cholesterol."

helicobacter pylori (H. pylori) – one of a large family of related bacteria that live in the stomachs of most vertebrates.

hemoglobin – a complex protein within red blood cells responsible for carrying oxygen to all other cells.

high blood pressure – hypertension; abnormally high blood pressure.

high-carbohydrate, low-fat diet – a diet that, because it is low in fat, is supposed to be good for weight loss.

homocysteine – a peptide that either promotes arteriosclerosis or is found in conjunction with arteriosclerosis; a potential risk factor for hardening of the arteries; a substance that is converted from emthionine, an amino acid.

hormone – a chemical released by an endocrine gland into the bloodstream that affects remote tissues and other hormones in specific ways.

human immunodeficiency virus (HIV) – the virus that leads to AIDS.

hydrogenation – the addition of hydrogen to an edible oil to convert it into a trans fat and saturated fat, usually solid at room temperature.

hypercholesterolemia – a condition characterized by an excess of cholesterol in the bloodstream.

hyperlipidemias – any condition characterized by an excess of fats in the bloodstream.

hyperthyroidism – overactivity of the thyroid gland, resulting in a rapid heartbeat and an increased rate of metabolism.

hypothyroidism – decreased activity of the thyroid gland.

idiopathic – of unknown cause.

immune response – activation of the immune system; ability of the body to protect against microbes, toxins, free radicals, and other threats.

immune system – a system of cells and proteins that protect the body from potential harm.

incidence – frequency; a statistical measure.

indigestion – difficulty in digesting food; pain or discomfort caused by this.

inflammation – redness, swelling, heat, and pain in a tissue due to injury or infection.

inflammatory bowel disease – chronic intestinal inflammation, including ulcerative colitis and Crohn's disease.

innocuous – harmless, non-toxic.

insomnia – the inability to sleep.

insulin – a polypeptide hormone produced in the pancreas by the islets of Langerhans, which regulates the amount of glucose in the blood, and the lack of which causes diabetes.

intestines − the principal part of the gastrointestinal tract, reaching from the exit of the stomach to the anus.

intravenous − within the blood circulation.

ischemia − blood starvation; oxygen deprivation resulting from inhibited blood flow.

Islets (or Islands) of Langerhans − small parts or globules of special cells (millions of them) within the pancreas. These islets secrete insulin and glucagons.

lactalbumin − a specific type of whey protein.

lactic acid − a carboxylic acid formed in the muscle tissues from glucose and glycogen during strenuous exercise.

lactobacillus acidophilus − a good bacteria present in the gut.

lactose − milk sugar.

lactose-intolerance − the inability to digest lactose accompanied by nausea, cramps, and diarrhea.

LDL cholesterol − low density lipoprotein (bad) cholesterol associated with increased risk of arteriosclerosis.

lesion − pathological area of tissue.

life process − a stage of life such as growth, puberty, or menopause.

lipids − fatty substances.

liver − the large, lobed, glandular organ in the abdomen, responsible for metabolizing fats, detoxifying, and neutralizing foreign and toxic substances.

Lou Gehrig's disease (ALS, or amyotrophic lateral sclerosis) − a rare, fatal, progressive, degenerative auto-immune disease of the nervous system that usually begins in middle age; characterized by increasing muscular weakness.

lupus − a chronic auto-immune disease causing inflammation of connective tissue.

lycopene − a carotenoid antioxidant found in brightly-coloured vegetables and fruits.

lymphocyte − a type of white blood cell crucial to the adaptive part of the immune system and made in the lymph nodes, bone marrow, and thymus gland; lymphocytes identify and "remember" invading disease organisms.

melatonin – a hormone produced in the body that helps us sleep.

membrane – a layer of usually very thin tissue that covers a bodily surface or forms some sort of barrier.

metabolism – all chemical processes taking place in the body; catabolic metabolism breaks down complex substances into simpler ones; anabolic metabolism manufactures complex substances from simple building blocks; the life process of a cell, which takes place in the mitochondria of the cell.

metabolize – to convert foods and other biochemicals into living bodily processes.

methionine – a thiol amino acid (sulphur containing).

migraine – an intermittent disorder of uncertain origin provoking vision disturbances, nausea, and severe, long-lasting headaches.

mitochondria – energy-generating component of cells.

modulate – to adjust in a controlled manner.

modulation – changing the amount of a substance; regulation of levels.

monosaccharides – a sugar that cannot be hydrolyzed to simpler carbo-hydrates of smaller carbon content. Glucose and fructose are examples.

monounsaturated fatty acids – fatty acids whose molecules contain one double bond in its carbon chain (contains one point of unsaturation).

mortality – death rate statistic.

motility – description of movement (e.g., food along intestinal tract).

multifactorial – having several causes or effects.

multiple sclerosis (MS) – a progressive, unpredictable disease of the nerv-ous system of auto-immune cause.

muscle – tissue consisting of elongated cells (muscle fibers) containing fib-rils that are highly contractile.

mycoplasma – types of microorganism without cell walls that are interme-diate between viruses and bacteria and are mostly parasitic.

myelin – fatty insulating sheath enclosing nerve fibers.

natural product – a substance found in nature as opposed to a pharma-ceutical product; also applied to substances found in nature but rendered to unnatural levels of concentration or purity.

naturopath – one who practices alternative medicine using a non-pharmaceutical approach.

negative feedback inhibition – balancing factor in which increased levels of a biochemical substance cause its continued secretion to slow down or stop.

nerve impulses – messages passed between the brain and various parts of the body through the nerves.

neural plaque formation – buildup of protein deposits in brain tissue and spinal cord.

neurodegenerative disorder – any progressive disease of the nervous system caused by physical and/or chemical changes of the brain and its chemical balance.

neurological – having to do with the brain and/or nervous system.

neuron – cell of the brain and nervous system.

neuropathy – disease, damage, or inflammation of peripheral nerves.

neurotransmitter – a chemical released from nerve endings that transmits information among neurons.

neutralize – to render ineffective; antioxidant donation of an electron to stabilize electrical charge.

non-food – any "food" that contains no life energy—few vitamins, minerals, fiber, or anything beneficial to sustain health; usually processed and packaged.

nutriceuticals – new term that describes therapies based on or including foods and food supplements.

nutritionist – health practitioner specializing in nutrition, alimentation, and absorption.

oral antioxidant supplements – concentrated food-like substances that help the body neutralize free radicals.

organic compounds – all compounds containing carbon except carbon oxides, carbon sulfides, and metal carbonates.

osteoporosis – loss of protein matrix tissue from bone, causing it to become brittle and to lose structural integrity.

over-training syndrome – negative effects on the body of excessive amounts or intensity of exercise.

oxidation – the normal process by which matter is metabolized to energy using oxygen.

oxidative stress – cellular and tissue damage resulting from oxidation and leading to bodily disorders.

oxidized glutathione (GSSG) – paired glutathione molecules that have neutralized free radicals by absorbing two negatively charged ions.

oxyradical – free radical; a molecule that through the natural process of oxidation is deprived of an electron and rendered toxic.

pancreas – a digestive organ/gland in the body that manufactures digestive enzymes as well as insulin and glucagons, hormones vital to the control of blood sugar levels in the body.

panic attack – a period of acute anxiety, sometimes focused on the fear of death or loss of reason.

paranoia – a delusion that certain persons or events are especially connected to oneself.

Parkinson's disease – shaking palsy; a neurological disorder characterized by muscular tremors, stiffness, and weakness and resulting in slow movement and a shuffling gait.

peer review – the rational and/or empirical scrutiny of published scientific reports by the scientific community at large.

peptide – a molecule made up of amino acids resembling a protein, but much smaller.

peristaltic – kneading or massaging, as in the action of the esophagus when pushing food down toward the stomach.

phospholipid – any of a group of fatty compounds composed of phosphoric esters, present in living cells (e.g., lecithin).

physiology – study of the physical and chemical processes of the cells, tissues, organs, and systems of the body; the foundation of all medical science.

phytates – compounds present in some foods that affect absorption of certain vitamins or minerals.

phytonutrients – plant chemicals beneficial to human health when ingested.

pituitary gland – the "master gland" situated in the brain that regulates and controls the activity of other endocrine glands and many body processes.

placebo – an inert substance used in controlled experiments against which the efficacy of a drug is compared.

plaque – a complex deposit of lipids, platelets, calcium, and scar tissue.

polyunsaturated fatty acids – any fatty acid molecule that contains more than one double bond in its carbon chain.

precursor – building block; usually simple proteins combined by the body into more complex molecules (e.g., glucose into glucosamine or beta-carotene into vitamin A).

predispose – to make particularly susceptible to or inclined towards a specific response.

preventive medicine – prevention of disease states by avoiding causes or conditions under which they develop.

prognosis – probable outcome of a disease process, taking into account the effectiveness of possible therapies.

programmed cell death – apoptosis; the self-destruction of cells initiated by outside causes.

prostaglandins – one of a group of fatty acid derivatives, originally identified in human prostate secretions but now known to be present in all tissues. Different prostaglandins often have opposite actions.

prostate cancer – a malignant growth in the outer part of the prostate gland; the most common cancer of men.

prostatic hyperplasia – an overgrowth of prostate tissue.

protein – fundamental component of the body; large molecule consisting of dozens to thousands of amino acids.

proteinuria – loss of protein in the urine.

psoriasis – a chronic skin condition characterized by inflammation and scaling.

psychosis − a severe disturbance of normal thought, perception, speech, and behaviour; mental disorder involving loss of contact with reality.

quercetin − a bioflavonoid.

radiotherapy − destruction of cells by radiation targeted at cancerous cells.

reactive metabolites − toxic products of normal metabolic oxidation.

reactive oxygen molecules − reactive oxygen species; compounds containing free oxygen radicals.

receptor − a biochemical docking bay on the surface of a cell that attracts certain molecules for specific purposes and enables the cell's activity to be influenced from the outside.

relapse − re-emergence or continued advance of disease after remission.

remission − the withdrawal or temporary halt of disease and its symptoms.

reperfusion − re-established blood flow, sometimes leading to reperfusion injury.

reperfusion injury − abnormal cellular function following reperfusion.

rheumatoid arthritis − systemic arthritis caused by an auto-immune disorder.

roughage − the indigestible portion of fibrous food.

sarcoidosis − a condition of auto-immune etiology leading to inflammation and scarring of tissues throughout the body.

saturated fatty acids − a fatty acid that contains no double bonds; present in almost all fats to some degree, but highest in animal fats.

schizophrenia − a chronic, severe, and disabling brain disease often causing patients to suffer symptoms such as hearing internal voices not heard by others, or believing that other people are reading their minds, controlling their thoughts, or plotting to harm them.

scientific study − investigation or research based on scientific principles of accounting and objectivity, open to peer review.

scurvy − a disease resulting from vitamin C deficiency.

selenium − a trace element found in meat, fish, whole grains, and dairy products.

sensorineural hearing loss − a problem of the inner ear or auditory nerve.

serotonin – a neurotransmitter (carries messages between nerve cells); works opposite to melatonin; serotonin is produced in response to increasing daylight to help you get out of bed in the morning.

shaking palsy – Parkinson's disease; a neurological disorder characterized by muscular tremors, stiffness, and weakness and resulting in slow movement and a shuffling gait.

sinusitis – inflammation or infection of the membranes lining the sinus cavities.

SLE – systemic lupus erythematosus (lupus); chronic inflammation of the connective tissue that holds body structures together.

smooth muscle – involuntary muscle of all internal organs; usually in the form of tubes or sheets, which may be several layers in thickness.

steroids – pharmaceutical corticosteroid drugs used against disease.

stomach ulcer – also called peptic ulcers; spots where the lining of the stomach has been eroded, leaving an open wound.

stress – physical, emotional, environmental, or biochemical pressure.

stroke – death of or damage to brain tissue resulting from blood deprivation.

sun lamp – electrical device that simulates sunlight, including ultraviolet radiation.

sustained release – a process like *timed release* (e.g., when consuming carbohydrates high in fiber, the sugars (carbohydrates) are released more slowly than if the food consumed had no fiber).

synergistic – the mutual enhancement of separate substances by which they enhance each other's efficacy.

synergy – when the sum of two or more substances, working together, is greater, or more beneficial, than if each of those substances were working separately.

thrush – an infection of the mouth or gullet by the fungus candida albicans.

tissue – a collection of cells specialized to perform a specific function.

toxicity – poisoning leading to impaired bodily function and/or cell damage.

trans fat – a fat that has been changed from its original form through either hydrogenation, heating, or other type of action; usually refers to poly- or monounsaturated fatty acids that have had their double bonds broken and hydrogen added.

trauma – the medical term for injury, usually referring to physical injury but also used to describe psychological injury.

tripeptide – a protein consisting of three amino acids.

tube feeding – nutrition supplied directly to the stomach or intestines.

ulcerative colitis (UC) – a chronic inflammatory disease of the mucous membranes of the colon leading to ulcers.

urethral passage – the path followed by urine from the bladder to the outside of the body.

urologist – physician specializing in disorders of the urinary tract.

vascular – pertaining to blood vessels.

vasculitis – inflammation of blood vessels.

vertebrae – individual bones of the spine.

vitamins – a group of complex nutrients not providing energy but essential in small amounts to the functioning of the body.

water-soluble – able to dissolve in water at normal temperature and pressure.

whey isolate protein – protein derived in highly pure concentrations from the liquid portion of cow's milk.

white blood cells – leukocytes (neutrophils, lymphocytes, and monocytes); cells that help protect the body against disease and infection; the main components of the immune system.

whole foods – any food that hasn't undergone changes by manufacturing or processing; a food that is as close as possible to its original, natural form.

xenobiotic – substance foreign to the body and/or biological processes, including infections and toxins.

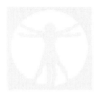

References

"Omega 3 Fatty Acids and their Impact on Cardiovascular Disease, Triglycerides, and Anti Inflammatory Actions." Presented by Dr. B. Holub, Department of Human Biology and Nutritional Sciences, University of Guelph, November 26, 2004.

Anesthesia. Edited by Ronald D. Miller. Third Edition. Churchill Livingstone, 1990.

Ascherio, A., C.H. Hennekens, J.E. Buring, C. Master, M.J. Stampfer, W.C. Willett. "Trans-fatty acids intake and risk of myocardial infarction." *Circulation 89* (1994): 94-101.

Balch, J.F. *The Antioxidant Revolution.* SoundConcepts, 2003.

Balch, James F., and Phyllis A. Balch. *Prescription for Nutritional Healing.* Avery Publishing Group, 1997.

Bateson-Koch, Carolee. *Allergies: Disease in Disguise.* Alive Books, 1994.

Brown, Marie-Annette, and Jo Robinson. *When Your Body Gets the Blues.* The Berkley Publishing Group, 2003.

Brudnak, Mark A. *The Probiotic Solution: Nature's Best-Kept Secret for Radiant Health.* Dragon Door Publications, Inc., 2003.

Campbell, T. Colin, with Thomas M. Campbell II. *The China Study.* Benbella Books, 2005.

Canfield, Jack, and Mark Victor Hansen. *Chicken Soup for the Soul: Living Your Dreams.* Health Communications, Inc., 2003.

Case, Shelley. *Gluten-Free Diet.* Case Nutrition Consulting, 2003.

Council for Responsible Nutrition. *The Benefits of Nutritional Supplements.* 2002.

d'Adamo, Peter J., and Catherine Whitney. *Eat Right 4 Your Type.* G.P. Putnam's Sons, 1996.

Davis, D., M. Epp, H. Riordan. "Changes in USDA Food Composition Data for 43 Garden Crops, 1950 to 1999." *Journal of the American College of Nutrition 23,* no. 6 (2004): 669-682.

De March, A. Kennel, M. De Bouwerie, M.N. Kolopp-Sarda, G.C. Faure, M.C. Béné, C.C.A. Bernard. "Anti-myelin olegodendrocyte B-cell responses in multiple sclerosis." *Journal of Neuroimmunology* 135 (2003): 117-125.

Dossey, Larry. *Healing Words: The Power of Prayer and the Practice of Medicine.* San Francisco: HarperSanFrancisco, 1993.

Embry, A. "Vitamin D and Seasonal Fluctuations of Gadolinium-Enhancing Magnetic Resonance Imaging Lesions in Multiple Sclerosis." *Annals of Neurology* 48, no. 2 (August 2000).

Embry, A. "Vitamin D Supplementation in the fight against multiple sclerosis." In personal communication to the author.

Erasmus, Udo. *Fats That Heal Fats That Kill.* Alive Books, 1997.

Fuller, DicQie. *The Healing Power of Enzymes.* Forbes Custom Publishing, 2002.

Gershoff, Stanley. *The Tufts University Guide to Total Nutrition.* Harper Perennial, 1996.

Gillie, O. "Sunlight Robbery: Health benefits of sunlight are denied by current public health policy in the UK." Health Research Forum 2004. Occasional Reports: No 1.

Graci, Sam. *The Food Connection.* Macmillan Canada, 2001.

Graham, Judy. *Multiple Sclerosis: A Self-Help Guide to Its Management.* Healing Arts Press, 1989.

Gray, John. *Mars and Venus Together Forever.* HarperPerennial, 1996.

Greenwood, Michael. *Braving the Void: Journeys into Healing.* PARADOX Publishers, 1997.

Greenwood, Michael. *The Unbroken Field: The Power of Intention in Healing.* Paradox Publishers, 2004.

Guggenmos, J., et al. "Antibody cross-reactivity between myelin oligodendrocyte glycoprotein and the milk protein butyrophilin in multiple sclerosis." *Journal of Immunology* (Oct. 2003).

Gutman, Jimmy. *GSH: Your Body's Most Powerful Protector GLUTATHIONE.* Montreal: FACEPCommunications Kudo.ca Inc., 2002.

Guyton, Arthur C. *Textbook of Medical Physiology.* W.B. Saunders Company, 1986.

Handbook of Clinical Nutrition and Aging. Edited by C. Watkins Bales and C. Seel Ritchie. Humana Press, 2004.

Harpe, Charls C. *GAC Juice Ancient Fruits Modern Powerhouse.* Sound Concepts Publishing, 2005.

Heo, H., and C. Lee. "Protective effects of quercetin and vitamin C against ouxidative stress–induced neurodegeneration." *Journal of Agricultural and Food Chemistry* 52, no. 25 (2004): 7514-7517.

Internal Medicine. Editor-in-Chief Jay H. Stein. Little, Brown and Company, 1983.

Jamison, Jennifer. *Clinical Guide to Nutrition & Dietary Supplements in Disease Management.* Churchill Livingstone, 2003.

Jelinek, George. *Taking Control of Multiple Sclerosis.* Hylan House Publishing Pty. Ltd., 2000.

Jonas, Wayne B., and Jeffrey S. Levin. *Essentials of Complementary and Alternative Medicine.* Lippincott Williams & Wilkins, 1999.

Kaye, Dennis. *Laugh, I thought I'd Die: My Life with ALS.* Penguin Books, 1994.

Kehoe, John. *Mind Power into the 21st Century.* Zoetic, Inc., 2004.

King, Brad J., and Michael A. Schmidt. *BIO-AGE Ten Steps to a Younger You.* Macmillan Canada, 2001.

Kraft, George H., and Marci Cantanzaro. *Living with Multiple Sclerosis: A Wellness Approach.* Demos Vermande, 1996.

Krause's Food, Nutrition & Diet Therapy. Edited by Lik Mahan and S. Escott-Stump. Elselvier, 2004.

Linington, R., U. Brehm, R. Egg, E. Dilitz, F. Deisenhamme, W. Poewe, L. Berger. "Antibodies against the myelin oligodendrocyte glycoprotein and the myelin basic protein in multiple sclerosis and other neurological diseases: A comparative study." *Brain* 122 (November 1999): 2047-2056.

Liu, B.A., M. Gordon, J.M. Labranche, T.M. Murray, R. Vieth, N.H. Shear. "Seasonal prevalence of vitamin D deficiency in institutionalized older adults." *Journal of the American Geriatrics Society* 45, no. 5 (1997): 598-603.

Lopez, A., et al. "Effect of emu oil on auricular inflammation induced with croton oil in mice." *American Journal of Veterinary Research* 60, no. 12 (1999): 1558-1561.

Losier, Michael J. *Law of ATTRACTION.* Michael J. Losier, 2003.

MacFarlane, Craig, with Gib Twyman. *Inner Vision.* Addax Publishing Group, 1997.

Mahan, L. Kathleen, and Sylvia Escott-Stump. *Food, Nutrition, & Diet Therapy.* Elsevier, 2004.

Majamaa, H., and E. Isolauri. "Probiotics: A novel approach in the management of food allergy." *Journal of Allergy and Clinical Immunology* 99, no. 2 (Feb 1997): 179-185.

Mana, P., M. Goodyear, C. Bernard, R. Tomioka, M. Freire-Garabal, D. Linares. "Tolerance induction by molecular mimicry: prevention and suppression of experimental autoimmune encephalomyelitis with the milk protein butyrophilin." *International Immunology* 16, no. 3 (Mar 2004): 489-499.

Margotta, Roberto. *An Illustrated History of Medicine.* The Hamlyn Publishing Group, 1967.

Maroon, J.C., and J.W. Bost. "Omega-3 fatty acids (fish oil as an anti-inflammatory: an alternative to nonsteroidal anti-inflammatory drugs for discogenic pain." *Surg Neurol* 65, no. 4 (Apr 2006): 326-331.

Marsh, Eva. *Black Patent Shoes: Dancing with MS.* Sideroad Press, 1996.

Mather, I., and L. Jacks. "A review of the molecular and cellular biology of butyrophilin, the major protein of bovine milk fat globule membrane." *Journal of Dairy Science* (1992).

Mathey, E., C. Breithaupt, A. Schubart, C. Linington. "Sorting the wheat from the chaff: identifying demyelinating components of the myelin oligodendrocyte glycoprotein (MOG)-specific autoantibody repertoire." *Eur. J. Immunol* 34 (2004): 2065-2071.

Moongkarndi, P., et al. "Antiproliferative activity of Thai medicinal plant extracts on human breast adenocarcinoma cell line." *Fitoterapia* 75 (2004): 375-377.

Morgan, Marlo. *Mutant Message from Forever.* HarperPerennial, 1999.

Mozaffarian, D., T. Pischon, S.E. Hankinson, et al. "Dietary intake of trans fatty acids and systemic inflammation in women." *American Journal of Clinical Nutrition* 79 (2004): 606-612.

Nakatani, K., et al. "Inhibotions of histamine release and prostaglandin E_2 syntheses by mangosteen, a Thai medicinal plant." *Biol Pharm Bull* 25, no. 9 (2002): 1137-1141.

Nakatani, K., T. Kuni, N. Kondo. "Arakawa Gamma mangostin inhibits inhibitor KB Kinase activity and decreases Lipopolysaccharide-Induced Cyclooxygenase-2 Gene Expression in C6 Rat Glioma Cells." *Mol Pharmacol* 66 (2004): 667-674.

O'Connor, Paul. *Multiple Sclerosis: The Facts You Need.* Key Porter Books, 1998.

Oeste, Heidi. *Never Give Up: Crofton's Lillian Postgate at 80.* Shalom Productions, Canada, 1999.

Ogg, S.L., A.K. Weldon, L. Dobbie, A.J. Smith, I.H. Mather. "Expression of butyrophilin (BTN 1a1) in lactating mammary gland is essential for the regulated secretion of milk-lipid droplets." *Proc Natl Acad Sci USA* 101, no. 27 (Jul 6, 2004): 10084-10089.

Ornish, Dean. *Reversing Heart Disease.* Ballantine Books, 1990.

Packer, Lester, and Carol Colman. *The Antioxidant Miracle.* John Wiley & Sons, Inc., 1999.

Politis, M.J., and A. Dmytrowich. "Promotion of Second Intention Wound healing by emu oil lotion. Comparative results with furasin, polysporin and cortisone Plast." *Reconstr. Surg.* 102 (1998): 2404-2407.

Polman, Chris H., Alan J. Thompson, T. Jock Murray, W. Ian McDonald. *Multiple Sclerosis: The Guide to Treatment and Management.* Demos Medical Publishing, Inc., 2001.

Potts, Phyllis. *Wheat-Free Cooking.* Beyond Words Publishing, 1998.

Prevention Magazine. *Food & Nutrition.* Edited by John Feltman. Rodale Press, Inc., 1993.

Reindl, M., et al. "Antibodies against the myelin oligodendrocyte glycoprotein and the myelin basic protein in multiple sclerosis and other neurological diseases: a comparative study." *Brain* 122 (1999): 2047-2056.

Roizen, Michael F. *Real Age: Are You as Young as You Can Be?* Realage, 1999.

Rosbo, K., et al. "Predominance of the autoimmune response to myelin oligodendrocyte glycoprotein (MOG) in multiple sclerosis: reactivity to the extracellular domain of MOG is directed against three main regions." *Eur J Immunol.* 27, no. 11 (1997 Nov): 3059-3069.

Rudin, Donald O., and Clara Felix with Constance Schrader. *The Omega-3 Phenomenon.* Collier Macmillan Canada, Inc., 1987.

Sarjeant, Doris, and Karen Evans. *Hard to Swallow.* Alive Books, 1999.

Sarno, John E. *Healing Back Pain.* Warner Books, 1991.

Schapiro, Randall T. *Symptom Management in Multiple Sclerosis.* Demos Medical Publishing Co., Inc., 1998.

Schneider, Meir, and Maureen Larkin with Dror Schneider. *The Handbook of Self-Healing.* Arkana Penguin Books, 1994.

Schneider, Meir. *Self-Healing: My Life and Vision.* Arkana/The Penguin Group, 1989.

Shafarman, Steven. *Awareness Heals: The Fledenkrais Method for Dynamic Health.* Perseus Books, 1997.

Simmie, Scott, and Julia Nunes. *The Last Taboo.* McClelland & Stewart Ltd., 2001.

Skinner, Henry Alan. *The Origin of Medical Terms.* Hafner Publishing Company, 1979.

Snowden, J.M., and M.W. Whitehouse. "Anti-inflammatory activity of emu oil in rats." *Inflammopharmacology* 5 (1997): 127-132.

Somersall, Allan C. *Nature's Goldmine: Harvesting Miracle Ingredients from Milk.* GOLDENeight Publishers, 2001.

Stefferl, A., et al. "Butyrophilin, a milk protein, modulates the encephalitogenic T cell response to myelin oligodendrocyte glycoprotein in experimental autoimmune encephalomyelitis." *J Immunol.* 165, no. 5 (2000 Sept 1): 2859-2865.

Stipanuk, M. *Biochemical and Physiological Aspects of Human Nutrition.* 2000.

The Oxford Medical Companion. Edited by John Walton, Jeremiah A. Barondess, and Stephen Lock. Oxford University Press, 1994.

Thompson, Lilian U., and Stephen C. Cunnane. *Flaxseed in Human Nutrition.* AOCS Press, 2003.

Thomson Healthcare. *PDR for Nutritional Supplements.* First Edition. Montvale, NJ: Medical Economics Company, Inc., 2001.

Tisserand, Robert. *Aromatherapy for Everyone.* London: Arkana, 1990.

Tolle, Eckhart. *The Power of NOW.* Namaste Publishing Inc., 1997.

Trang, H.M., D.E. Cole, L.A. Rubin, A. Pierratos, S. Siu, R. Vieth. "Evidence that vitamin D_3 increases serum 25-hydroxyvitamin D more efficiently than does vitamin D_2." *Am J. Clin. Nutr.* 68, no. 4 (1998): 854-858.

Vacaleri, Franco. *Potential Within: A Guide to Nutritional Empowerment.* Biologic Publishing, Inc., 2003.

Vander Aa, A., N. Hellings, C.C. Bernard, J. Rous, P. Stinssen. "Functional properties of myelin oligodendrocyte glycoprotein – reactive T in multiple sclerosis of patients and controls." *J Neuroimmunol.* 137, no. 1-2 (2003): 164-176.

Vander Mei, I., A. Ponsonby, L. Blizzard, T. Dwyer. "Regional variation in Multiple Sclerosis prevalence in Australia and its association with ambient Ultraviolet radiation." *Neuroepidemiology* 20, no. 3 (2001 Aug): 168-174.

Vander Mei, I., A. Ponsonby, L. Blizzard, T. Dwyer. "Regional variation in Multiple Sclerosis prevalence in Australia and its association with ambient ultraviolet radiation." *Neuroepidemiology* 20, no. 3 (2001 Aug): 168-174.

Vanderhaeghe, Lorna R. *Healthy Immunity*. Macmillan Canada, 2001.

Vieth, R. "Vitamin D nutrition and its potential health benefits for bone, cancer and other conditions." *J. Envir. and Nut. Med.* 11.4.15 (2001).

Vieth, R. *The Pharmacology of Vitamin D, Including Fortification Strategies*. Edited by Feldman. Glorieux & Pike, 2004.

Vieth, R., R. Chan Pak-Cheung, G. MacFarlane. "Efficacy and safety of vitamin D_3 intake exceeding the lowest observed adverse effect level." *Am J Clin Nutr* 73 (2001): 288-294.

Walford, Roy. *Beyond the 120 Year Diet*. Four Walls Eight Windows, 2000.

Weil, Andrew. *Eating Well for Optimum Health*. New York: Alfred A. Knoph, 2000.

Weissert, R., et al. "High immunogenuicity of intracellular myelin oligodendrocyte glycoprotein epitopes." *J Immunol.* 169, no. 1 (2002 July 1): 548-556.

Willet, W.C., M.J. Stampfer, J.E. Mason, et al. "Intake of trans fatty acids and risk of coronary heart disease among women." *Lancet* 341 (1993): 581-585.

Williams, Montel, and Wini Linguvic. *Body Change*. Mountain Movers Press, 2001.

Worwood, Valerie Ann. *The Fragrant Pharmacy*. Bantam Books, 1993.

Zemach-Bersin, David, Kaethe Zemach-Bersin, and Mark Reese. *Relaxercise: The Easy New Way to Health and Fitness*. HarperSanFrancisco, 1990.

Index

ABOUT THE AUTHORS

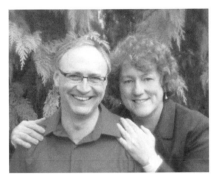

Bill Code, MD, has been involved in the field of medicine since 1975, maintaining a thriving practice until being diagnosed with painful multiple sclerosis. This turn of events set him on a new course of study, which contributed ultimately to reversing his MS symptoms and allowing him to reclaim his life. He now successfully applies traditional medicine with scientifically based alternative approaches to assist people with pain and chronic disease management. In 2006 Dr. Code was accepted for a Fellowship in Integrative Medicine at the University of Arizona under Dr. Andrew Weil & Associates. This has allowed him to further his goal of enhancing his expertise in treating pain and brain issues from an integrative approach.

Denise Code, MSc, RD, holds a Master's Degree in Nutrition and is a vital partner with her husband, Dr. Bill, in the research and application of what they are continually discovering in the areas of brain and stroke research, nutrition, and physiology. She has been by his side in both his personal challenge with MS and in his professional work.

Dr. Bill and Denise Code live near Vancouver, Canada, though they travel extensively lecturing on leading-edge discoveries in pain relief and working with chronic illness. They are dedicated to assisting patients and pain sufferers to get the most out of medical and natural treatments. Bill and Denise have three grown, college-graduate children, of whom they are very proud.

WWW.DRBILLCODE.COM